Day Surgery
Contemporary Approaches to Nursing Care

Edited By

Dr Fiona Timmins

Senior Lecturer
School of Nursing and Midwifery, Trinity College Dublin
Ireland

And

Ms Catherine McCabe

Lecturer
School of Nursing and Midwifery, Trinity College Dublin
Ireland

WILEY-BLACKWELL
A John Wiley & Sons, Ltd., Publication

This edition first published 2009
© 2009 John Wiley & Sons, Ltd.

Wiley-Blackwell is an imprint of John Wiley & Sons, formed by the merger of Wiley's global Scientific, Technical and Medical business with Blackwell Publishing.

Registered office
John Wiley & Sons Ltd, The Atrium, Southern Gate, Chichester,
West Sussex, PO19 8SQ, United Kingdom

Editorial office
John Wiley & Sons Ltd, The Atrium, Southern Gate, Chichester,
West Sussex, PO19 8SQ, United Kingdom

For details of our global editorial offices, for customer services and for information about how to apply for permission to reuse the copyright material in this book please see our website at www.wiley.com/wiley-blackwell.

The right of the author to be identified as the author of this work has been asserted in accordance with the Copyright, Designs and Patents Act 1988.

Wiley also publishes its books in a variety of electronic formats. Some content that appears in print may not be available in electronic books.

Designations used by companies to distinguish their products are often claimed as trademarks. All brand names and product names used in this book are trade names, service marks, trademarks or registered trademarks of their respective owners. The publisher is not associated with any product or vendor mentioned in this book. This publication is designed to provide accurate and authoritative information in regard to the subject matter covered. It is sold on the understanding that the publisher is not engaged in rendering professional services. If professional advice or other expert assistance is required, the services of a competent professional should be sought.

Library of Congress Cataloguing-in-Publication Data

Day surgery : contemporary approaches to nursing care / edited by Fiona
Timmins and Catherine McCabe.
p. ; cm.
Includes bibliographical references and index.
ISBN 978-0-470-31984-0 (pbk. : alk. paper)
1. Ambulatory surgical nursing. I. Timmins, Fiona, 1967– II. McCabe, Catherine.
[DNLM: 1. Ambulatory Surgical Procedures–nursing. 2. Ambulatory Surgical
Procedures–trends. 3. Patient Education as Topic. 4. Perioperative Nursing.
WY 161 D2745 2009]

RD110.5.D39 2009
617'.024–dc22
2008027936

A catalogue record for this book is available from the British Library.

Set in 10 on 12 pt Sabon by SNP Best-set Typesetter Ltd., Hong Kong
Printed in Singapore by Fabulous Printers Pte Ltd
1 2009

Contents

Contributors

Ms Anne-Marie Brady
Lecturer
School of Nursing and Midwifery
Trinity College Dublin
Ireland.

Ms Sharon Farlow
Theatre Service Manager, Bishop Auckland General
Hospital/Darlington Memorial Hospital County Durham and Darlington
NHS Foundation Trust, UK.

Dr Jo Gilmartin
School Of Health Care Studies
Baines Wing, University of Leeds
Leeds, UK.

Ms Catherine McCabe
Lecturer
School of Nursing and Midwifery
Trinity College Dublin
Ireland.

Ms Margaret McCann
Lecturer
School of Nursing and Midwifery
Trinity College Dublin
Ireland.

Professor Robert McSherry
Professor Nursing and Practice Development
Practice Development Team
School of Health and Social Care
University of Teesside, Middlesbrough, UK.

Ms Kay Scott
Senior Lecturer
School of Health and Social Care
University of Teesside
Middlesbrough, UK.

Dr Fiona Timmins
Senior Lecturer
School of Nursing and Midwifery
Trinity College Dublin
Ireland.

Ms Phillipa Ryan Withero
Nurse Practice Development Coordinator
Adelaide Meath incorporating the National Children's Hospital
(AMNCH)
Tallaght, Dublin
Ireland.

Introduction to Day Surgery

Phillipa Ryan Withero

Historical background

The evolution of day surgery has heralded a new era of medical, anaesthetic and nursing knowledge, skills and practice. Surgical techniques and techno-logical advances coupled with developments in anaesthetic approaches have contributed positively and significantly not only to the initial but ongoing developments within the field of day surgery, which today accounts for 50–80% of all surgical procedures. The international drive to increase day surgery rates is grounded in the well articulated benefits including: reduced demand for overnight or weekend staff, hence reduced costs; more rapid throughput of patients; reduction in the number of patients on waiting lists and reduction in the number of patients who fail to attend for surgery. Potential problems associated with surgery (post-operative nausea, vomiting or pain), responsibility for which may fall within a self-care remit or entail an increased burden on community services, require attention to ensure that day surgery services appropriately address these requirements. The political, economic and policy-driven demands for greater bed utilisation, value for money and cost containment measures have influenced the expansion and development of day surgery throughout its history.

The growth of day surgery, albeit a substantial one, is not a new concept. In the early stages of nursing, its founder, Florence Nightingale, noted that patients should not stay a day longer than is absolutely necessary in all hospitals and in particular children's hospitals (Nightingale 1914). In recog-nising the significant value a shorter hospital stay has for the patient, her opinion was not based upon economic or political perspectives, but on reducing the possibility of patients contracting further illness or diseases as a result of hospitalisation.

One of the earliest references to day surgery is that of the now landmark publication by Dr Nicoll in the *British Medical Journal* in 1909. Nicoll outlined his ten-year surgical experience of performing 8988 day surgery procedures at a Glasgow outpatients clinic for sick children. Over half of the children were less than three years old. The procedures included treatment of cleft palate, hare lip, hernias, talipes and mastoid diseases. Nicoll disapproved of hospitalisation and was adamant that children should return to their nursing mothers as early as possible. Even at this early stage of day surgery, he drew attention to the necessity for suitable home conditions in addition to General Practitioner (GP) support, a feature that was reiterated in 1955 by Farquharson.

In 1916 Ralph Waters wrote about his establishment of a free-standing anaesthesia clinic in Iowa, providing day surgery for dental and minor surgery cases. The revolution had begun. Hospital-based ambulatory units were developed in 1959 by Webb and Horace in Vancouver, in 1962 by Cohen and Dillon in Los Angeles and in 1970 by Levy and Coakley in Washington. The first successful free-standing ambulatory facility was established in 1969 by Ford and Reed in Arizona (Epstein 2005).

The day surgery revolution within the United Kingdom (UK) was slower to progress since first being mooted by Nicoll in 1909. It was not until over 50 years later, in 1960, that the first stand-alone day surgery unit within a hospital in the UK was developed at Hammersmith (Calnan and Martin 1971). In response to the evolution of day surgery, the Royal College of Surgeons in England published *Guidelines for Day Surgery* in 1985, based upon a working party report which stated that day surgery was the best possible option for 50% of all patients undergoing surgical procedures electively. At the time of the report the national average for day surgery was as low as 15%, despite Palumbo et al. (1952) outlining the possibility of greater bed utilisation owing to a shorter length of stay.

In 1989 the British Association of Day Surgery was established with a multidisciplinary membership, recognising the necessity for quality in the delivery of day surgery and the potential benefits, not only for patients but for the health service. Key drivers for day surgery within the UK were a number of pivotal reports published over a short period of time, which brought into intense focus the proliferation of day surgery units and facilities within the National Health Service (NHS). The first of these, the Bevan Report (1989), was undertaken by the NHS Management Executive Value for Money Unit. Support for day surgery expansion was indicated, given the significant impact it would have on waiting lists and financial costs. In 1990 the Audit Commission, an external auditor for the NHS, published *A Short Cut to Better Services*. This report is now recognised as one of the major catalysts for the development and advancement of day surgery within the UK. It examined the expansion of day surgery within England and

Wales, concluding that the rate of expansion was slower than anticipated; it also identified significant variances in day surgery between health authorities. A consequence of the report was the introduction of what became known as the 'basket' of 20 common procedures – still in use today – that could be performed as day surgery cases. The rationale for the introduction of this 'basket' of procedures was to develop uniformity and limit the variance in day surgery procedures across the health service, with a view to improving cost-effectiveness by increasing the number of patients that could be treated as day cases. The Audit Commission also reported on possible barriers to the growth of day surgery, such as lack of facilities, poor management structures and a preference for traditional approaches, and suggested methods to overcome them.

Building on the Audit Commission report, in 1991 the Value for Money Unit published *Day Surgery: Making it Happen*. This report focused on the design, practice and management of day units, outlined recommendations on staffing, training and quality, and highlighted the financial rewards for the NHS. Also in 1991 the Audit Commission reported on day surgery from the patient's perspective: their investigation found that 80% of patients preferred day case surgery, with 83% recommending this approach to a friend. This report reinforced awareness of acceptance of day surgery by patients, thus justifying the continued expansion of this approach to surgery.

One of the motivating factors for the expansion of day surgery was clearly the resultant financial rewards for the NHS, although significant funding for the establishment of day surgery facilities would first be required. In recognition of the financial implications, a regional task force to oversee investment was established in the early 1990s. The task force produced a toolkit for managers and clinicians as an aid for the establishment and review of day surgery facilities, and set a target of 50% for all elective surgery as day case procedures. Despite significant investment, the report of the task force in 1993 revealed that few proposals had been implemented, with considerable variation in progress towards meeting the 50% target across the NHS, and raised the target to 75%. Not surprisingly, in 2001 the Audit Commission confirmed that no service was achieving 75%, with a number of units not being utilised to maximum capacity. Consequently, £31 million was invested from the Funding treasury Capital Modernisation in order to achieve the target of 75%. In conjunction with the launch of the Day Surgery Strategy in 2002, the *Day Surgery Operational Guide* was published in order to support the drive towards achieving the target of 75% and the Department of Health's commitment to this strategy was evidenced by the inclusion of day surgery for inpatient stays as one of the NHS Modernisation Agency's '10 High Impact Changes'.

By 2003 the Healthcare Commission was created and given the authority to take over responsibilities from other commissions, including the Audit Commission. In a review of the acute hospital day surgery portfolio in 2005, the Healthcare Commission reported that variability in the organisation of day surgery continued to exist. Determining the overall achievement of the 75% target proved difficult as a result of this variability. The report concluded that support for increased capacity and measures to improve the level of uptake of day surgery should be continued.

Approaches to day surgery development vary within the developed world. The Republic of Ireland (ROI), for example, although in close proximity to the UK, presents a very different picture in terms of progression and innovation: the motivation towards an increase in day surgery rates in ROI was much slower and less well defined. The reasons for this are multifaceted and include complex factors related to gross under-funding of the health system in addition to organisation, management and structure of the health system itself. In 1980 day surgery rates were as low as 2%, which is not surprising given that the number of day surgery beds recorded for that period was just 26 (DOHC 2002). In the period between 1980 and 2000, this figure increased to 562, with a subsequent increase in overall activity from 2% to 38%. The low level of day surgery rates in Ireland in the 1980s was indicative of significant under-funding of services during this period. The 1990s saw a period of reform in which the Irish healthcare system was struggling to compensate for the investment deficit of the 1980s. The most significant increase in day surgery rates occurred during the decade 1990–99, when figures rose from 20% of total activity to 38% (DOHC 2002). Much of the early developments and achievements can be attributed to the health strategy of 1994, 'Shaping a Healthier Future' (DOHC 1994).

One of the earliest references promoting the advancement of day surgery in ROI was made by the Report of the Commission on Health Funding (1989), which highlighted the cost-effectiveness of increased bed utilisation in the context of the lengthy waiting lists which were a feature of healthcare at this period. Concluding that an improvement in the utilisation of hospital beds as a result of day surgery would positively impact on waiting lists, the report recommended the development and implementation of a 'casemix' funding approach, which would lead to a rapid move towards the provision of surgery on an outpatient or day ward basis. This recommendation was a major catalyst in the development of day surgery in Ireland: funding was awarded on the basis of increased bed utilisation and activity and the National Casemix programme was instituted in 1991 (DOHC 2004). A national review of the casmix programme in 2004, 12 years following its institution, concluded that 95% of all acute inpatient and day-case hospital admissions were participating in the national casemix programme, with 20% of the activity related funding for the hospitals being casemix dependent (DOHC 2004).

In a number of governmental reports, which strengthened efforts to progress day surgery by reinforcing the benefits of this approach, a common theme was the absence of clearly defined national targets for day surgery rates in Ireland. The impetus for improvement in day surgery rates appeared to rely on the motivation to procure additional funding through the casemix programme, based upon day surgery performance activity rates. The 1994 health strategy, 'Shaping a Healthier Future', outlined the significant increase in day surgery rates, from 15% in 1987 to 25% in 1993, and indicated the expected rise in this trend for the years ahead. Specific, quantifiable targets for improvement in day surgery rates were not, and are still not clearly articulated, with performance assessment based solely upon the impact on hospital waiting lists.

Healthcare waiting lists endured as a constant feature within the Irish healthcare system. In 1998 the report of the review group on the waiting list initiative recommended a continued move towards day case work (DOHC 1998) and proposed a close examination for the provision of stand-alone day surgery units on acute hospital sites in order to address the number of patients on waiting lists between 1999 and 2001.

Acknowledged within the report was the necessity, as a matter of urgency, to review and address the capacity of acute hospitals. The contentious issue of hospital capacity is one that was mirrored by the value for money audit of the Irish healthcare system by Deloitte and Touche (DOHC 2001a). The audit, commissioned by the Department of Health, concluded that although day surgery rates were improving, overall capacity of the acute hospitals was adversely affecting bed utilisation in addressing the significant waiting list. Utilisation of day surgery beds for inpatient care was a becoming a common feature as a direct result of capacity issues within the acute hospital sector. The publication of the health strategy *Quality and Fairness* (DOHC 2001b) sought to address these issues. This report focused on equitable access to service and set as one of its targets an increase in proportion the number of one-day procedures. Although it did not quantify this increase in terms of a national target, it did recommend the establishment of a National Treatment Purchase Fund, whereby patients on the public waiting list could avail themselves of treatment purchased by the state from private hospitals. Since its establishment in April 2002, the NTPF has facilitated 120,000 cases/people (www.ntpf.ie accessed September 2008). The impact on the public service has been to relieve the capacity crisis by reducing the number of day-case beds being inappropriately used as inpatient beds, so reducing the number of patients on hospital waiting lists. The organisational and structural components of the health system also required attention in order to drive these changes.

The Health Service Reform Programme (DOHC 2003) outlined the structural changes that were necessary in order achieve positive improvement in healthcare delivery in Ireland. These included rationalisation and reorganisation of the existing health service agencies to reduce fragmentation, and the establishment of a Health Service Executive on the basis of three core divisions: a National Hospitals Office; a Primary Community and Continuing Care Directorate; and a National Shared Services Centre. The National Hospitals Office is now charged with the responsibility for the management of the acute hospitals sector.

As a result of these reports, strategies and reforms, the number of day-case procedures in Ireland has continued to rise annually, from 357,676 cases in 2001 to 448,676 cases in 2003 (DOHC 2005). The importance of governmental policy in supporting the development of day-case approaches to surgery should not be underestimated. Advances in anaesthesia, surgical technique and nursing care in day surgery require significant financial, managerial and organisational support, not only at a high level within an organisation but also at governmental policy level, in order to establish a coordinated and committed approach. Although the rate of development of day surgery care may vary between countries and within national health care provision, what is important is the obvious benefit not only for providers but also for patients.

Overview of services

Day surgery services are constantly evolving and are delivered in a variety of ways in a variety of units. In order to gain the insight required to interpret them in detail, it is pertinent to examine specifics such as how and where services are delivered and levels of patient satisfaction achieved; definitions, terminology, structure, organisation and delivery of day care also require exploration.

Traditionally day surgery is defined as the same-day admission and discharge for a planned surgical procedure whereby the patient has made a complete recovery from their procedure. The patient may undergo a pre-assessment procedure whereby their suitability for day surgery will be assessed. The term 'ambulatory surgery' is used interchangeably to describe the same process. There are a variety of ways to provide ambulatory/ day surgery services, each with its advantages and disadvantages.

Office or outpatient surgery

Day surgery operations or procedures carried out in the medical practitioner's own office or outpatient department, by their very nature, do not require treatment or observation in a day surgery centre or unit. This type of service offers patients swift access to minor surgical procedures, without the necessity for admission or observation (IAAS 2003; Australian Day Surgery Council 2004).

Free-standing day surgery centre or day surgery facility

Free-standing day surgery centres are self-contained units designed solely for day surgery, which ultimately result in greater patient satisfaction rates

(DH 2002; Seibert et al. 1999), typically contain their own admission unit and clinical, theatre and recovery areas. Although the initial development costs are high, these units prove to be the most cost-effective option long-term (Bureau of Health Planning and Resources Development 1997), because they offer a more streamlined approach to the patient's surgical journey. A noteworthy disadvantage of these facilities is their limited access to broader services, such as intensive care and radiology, which may be necessary as a result of unforeseen complications in the post-operative period (Cahill and Jackson 1997). This is an issue specifically addressed in emerging guidelines and standards, whereby some such units will need to have immediate access to facilities for unforeseen major complications (Australian Day Surgery Council 2004). Dedicated teams solely employed by these facilities are necessary, as movement of staff, in particular of surgeons between healthcare facilities has the potential to reduce the efficiency of day surgery centres.

Dedicated day surgery and shared day surgery facilities within a hospital

Dedicated day surgery facilities are purpose-built units within an existing hospital, with their own admission suite, theatre, recovery and discharge areas. This type of unit is the most desirable, as it operates independently of the hospital but has the considerable advantage of immediate access to facilities such as radiology and intensive care or inpatient admission in the event of unforeseen complications. Shared day surgery facilities within a hospital denotes the establishment of a day surgery facility with separate admission, pre-assessment and clinical areas but shared theatre and recovery areas. The advantage of this type of facility is the separation of inpatient and day-patient activity. A dedicated pre-assessment area within the unit offers patients not only the advantage of familiarity with the unit's geography but also the opportunity to meet the clinical staff who will be caring for them. Disadvantages include sharing of recovery and theatre space; in particular the latter may lead to an increase in day surgery cancellations in favour of inpatient lists; day surgery patients may also be delayed until later in the daily theatre list, resulting in a later discharge or the risk of cancellation and unplanned overnight admission.

Parallel day surgery facility within a hospital

In this type of unit, day surgery patient admission, theatre and recovery are all carried out in parallel to existing in-patient services. The patient in this unit is at a significant disadvantage in comparison to the previously described units: the possibilities for delay at the point of entry, cancellation or even admission overnight, are enhanced. In comparison to a free-standing unit, the increase in the rate of overnight admissions rises from 2.4% to 14% (Cahill and Tillin 1995). Moreover, the complex nature of some patients' demands in the clinical area requires increased nursing-care time, limiting the level of attention available for less complex day surgery patients. One great advantage of this type of facility is that they are less costly to establish.

Extended day surgery facility

Some services have developed extended day surgery facilities. These may be purpose-built, free-standing, or within a day surgery centre or hospital specifically designed for purposes of extended recovery from day surgery procedures. Extended recovery includes any admission and discharge within 23 hours. Once the 23-hour period is exceeded, the patient is no longer a day-case patient and is classed as an inpatient. One key advantage of this type of facility is the ability to perform complex major surgical cases, which are suitable as day surgery but require an extended period of recovery not exceeding 23 hours. These facilities also permit evening surgery, facilitating recovery and discharge the following day within the 23-hour period, rather than discharge at an unsociable hour. One potential challenge is that surgeons and patients may choose to avail of an optional overnight stay which may not be absolutely necessary, thus leading to an overall reduction in reported day surgery rates. One way to address this difficulty is to separate fully day surgery and extended day surgery facilities. However, in practice this is not practical or feasible, as it would mean separation of clinical expertise rather than concentration and cohesion of clinical expertise at one site. The cost of overnight staffing also requires careful examination in the choice of this facility.

Limited care accommodation

This innovative initiative includes accommodating day surgery patients in hospital, hotel or hostel accommodation, where professional healthcare is available on an on-call basis. This type of accommodation is also utilised to support patients requiring a longer stay due to social rather than medical/ nursing needs. As this is a new concept in day surgery, there is as yet little evidence to demonstrate its effectiveness or its limitations. The Australian Day Surgery Council report recommendations on the use of this type of facility include: physician-only determination of patient suitability; connected to or on-site with the acute hospital; immediate availability of a manager or attendant, such as a nurse or person trained in CPR; an emergency 24-hour call system in the room; CPR trolley; medical utility room, arrangements for immediate transfer to an acute hospital; and appropriate records (Australian Day Surgery Council 2004).

Whatever the service location or type, the quality of the service delivery to patients is of paramount importance. Within the realm of day surgery services, quality is high on the agenda, with numerous reviews and research initiatives on the efficacy of this approach to surgery from the patient's perspective, utilising patient satisfaction levels as a clinical indicator of service delivery. In conjunction with the development of day surgery in the UK, the Audit Commission and later the Healthcare Commission completed a number of reviews of day surgery in the NHS to ascertain patient satisfaction with the delivery of this service (Audit Commission 2001; Healthcare Commission 2005).

Today's Day surgery units are providing improved outcomes for both patient care and indeed satisfaction as a direct result of process improvements in a number of key areas such as: patient pre-assessment within six weeks of admission; choice of appointments at the booking phase; individualised patient arrival times; telephone reminders about admission date and time to patients; pre-admission and discharge written information; all of these initiatives have positively resulted in a reduction in non-attenders (Healthcare Commission, 2005).

Additional key indicators of patient satisfaction in day surgery are the management of post-operative pain, nausea and vomiting. Post-operative pain control is a prominent and well documented feature in surgery and, indeed, within day surgery (Yeng et al. 2002). Within day-case surgery, several studies have demonstrated an association of well managed post-operative pain control, nausea and vomiting with increased levels of patient satisfaction (Jenkins et al. 2001; Gan et al. 2001; Bain et al. 1999; Scott and Hodson 1997). Overall day surgery is viewed positively not only from the health service providers' perspective but – more importantly – from the patients' perspective.

Common presenting conditions

The scope of day surgery procedures has steadily expanded since the initial concept was described. By the end of the twentieth century, day surgery procedures had increased profoundly, with significant growth in the number of facilities offering treatment. The largest influencers of day surgery practice and, more essentially, procedures include governmental organisations, national and international dedicated day surgery associations, and colleges of surgery.

From an international perspective, the International Association for Ambulatory Surgery has completed regular, ongoing surveys of day surgery procedures, in an attempt to define the categories not only of common procedures but also of revolutionary procedures. As already mentioned, in collaboration with the Association, De Lathouwer and Pouiller (1998) conducted two surveys, in 1994 and 1996, defining a 'basket' of 20 procedures. The International Association for Ambulatory Surgery undertook a further survey in 2003 (IAAS 2003), in which the original 20 procedures were supplemented by 17 more. This increase in procedures has occurred primarily due to an increase in the number of surgical specialities, such as vascular and urology, in addition to developments of surgical procedures suitable for day case surgery. These include laparoscopic assisted hysterectomy and Trans Urethral Resection of the Prostate (TURP). Table 1.1 lists

Table 1.1 Surgical procedures suitable for day case surgery I (*IAAS 2003*)

Procedure	Specialty
Cataract removal	*Opthalmology*
Squint correction	
Myringotomy with tube insertion	*Ear, Nose and Throat*
Tonsillectomy	
Rhinoplasty	
Surgical removal of tooth	*Dental*
Endoscopic female sterilization	*Gynaecology*
Termination of pregnancy	
Dilatation and curettage of uterus	
Hysterectomy	
Inguinal hernia	*General surgery and Urology*
Circumcision	
Orchidectomy + – Orchidepexi	
Male sterilisation	
Varicose veins	
Pilonidal sinus	
Transurethral resection of the prostate	
Knee arthroscopy	*Orthopaedics*
Arthroscopic meniscus	
Removal of bone implants	
Repair of deformity on foot	
Carpel tunnel release	
Baker cyst	
Dupuytrens contracture	
Cruciate ligament repair	
Disc operations	
Repair of cysto and rectocele	*General surgery*
Local excision of breast	
Mastectomy	
Laparoscopic cholecystectomy	
Laparoscopic anti-reflux	
Haemorrhiodectomy	
Broncho-mediasinoscopy	
Bilateral breast reduction	*Plastic Surgery*
Abdominoplasty	
Removal of colon polyps	*Endoscopic*
Colonoscopy with/without biopsy	

these procedures and their respective specialities from the International Association of Ambulatory Surgery (IAAS 2003).

In the UK, a 'basket' of procedures was similarly developed over 15 years ago, outlining 20 procedures suitable for day surgery (Audit Commission 1990). This list has been recently reviewed in association with the British Association of Day Surgery and now constitutes 25 procedures upon which current day surgery performance in the NHS is based. This new set of 25 procedures details a list of common procedures in addition to those that may be suitable for day case surgery (Healthcare Commission 2005). Table 1.2 outlines the list of 25 procedures (Healthcare Commission 2005).

Within the Republic of Ireland, determining an exact 'basket' or list of procedures presents significant difficulty, as a result of the aforementioned casemix approach to recording clinical cases. The reporting of day-case procedures via the casemix method records the total number of day cases by case groups which includes day case chemotherapy, radiation, transfusions etc which are clearly not day surgical procedures. Moreover whereby procedures are recorded it is as a grouping procedure rather than a statement of the actual procedure. As a result extrapolation of this data from

Table 1.2 Surgical procedures suitable for day case surgery II (*IAAS 2003*)

Procedure	Speciality
Extract of cataract with/without implant	*Opthalmology*
Correction of squint	
Myringotomy	*Ear, Nose and Throat*
Tonsillectomy	
Sub mucous resection	
Reduction of nasal fracture	
Operation for bat ears	
Dilatation and curettage/hysteroscopy	*Gynaecology*
Laparoscopy	
Termination of pregnancy	
Carpel tunnel decompression	*Orthopaedics*
Excision of ganglion	
Arthroscopy	
Bunion operations	
Removal of metalware	
Excision of Dupuytren's contracture	
Orchidopexy	*General surgery and Urology*
Circumcision	
Inguinal hernia repair	
Excision of breast lump	
Anal fissure dilatation or excision	
Haemorrhiodectomy	
Laparoscopic cholecystectomy	
Varicose vein stripping or ligation	
Transurethral resection of bladder tumour	

the casemix groups was required to generate the following list of procedures in Table 1.3 (DOHC 2005).

Instituting a nationally agreed set of procedures has significant advantages, which include: standardised safe approaches to practice and procedures; clarity on the scope of suitable day procedures and revolutionary procedures being undertaken; evaluation and review of performance relative to national and international targets, with a clear vision on the direction of

Table 1.3   Surgical procedures suitable for day case surgery III (*DOHC, 2005*)

Procedure	Speciality
Eye procedures	*Opthalmology*
Internal ear procedures	*Ear, Nose and Throat*
ENT procedures	
Nasal procedures	
Sinus procedures	
Tonsil/adenoid/gland procedures	
Tympanoplasty	
Dental surgery	*Dental*
Gynaecological and peritoneal procedures	*Gynaecology*
Aspirations and endoscopic gynaecological procedures	
Evacuations	
Spinal procedures	*Orthopaedics*
Knee procedures	
Hand and foot procedures	
Lower limb procedures	
Upper limb procedures	
Elbow procedures	
Open reduction and fusion	
Removal of internal orthopaedic devices	
Tendon and muscle procedures	
Soft tissue procedures	
Closed reduction	
Other bone procedures	
Maxillo-facial procedures	*Plastic Surgery*
Vascular procedures	*General surgery and Urology*
Lower urinary tract procedures	
Upper urinary tract procedures	
Ano-rectal procedures	
Male genital procedures	
Cholecystectomy	
Trans-urethreal prostatectomy	
Lithotripsy	
Mastectomy	
Circumcision	
Hepato-biliary procedures	
Hernia procedures	
Plastic procedures	
Breast plastic procedure	

day surgery. Management and organisation of day surgery in this approach also facilitates greater understanding and knowledge by patients, with enhanced clarity on exact day surgery procedures and of the day surgery facilities offered within their health service. This approach offers health-care providers the opportunity to compare their individual services based upon an agreed procedure list, in order to identify areas for process improvement.

Recent innovations in day surgery

The rapid expansion of day surgery as a result of surgical, technological and anaesthetic advances has demanded equal advancement in nursing practice. Pioneering nursing roles and practices as a specialty within day surgery have emerged in response to these developments. In particular, these advances have signalled the development of nurse-led pre-assessment clinics for patients attending for day surgery (Hilditch et al. 2003a; Hilditch et al. 2003b; Fellowes et al. 1999; Dunn 1998), which will be further discussed in Chapter Three. This initiative has signalled the development of nursing education programmes specifically designed for pre-assessment skills in conjunction with guidelines for practice (NHS Modernisation Agency 2002; Ormrod and Casey 2004). One of the criticisms of nurse-led pre-assessment in day surgery is that it is medically driven and consisting of tasks (Rai and Pandit 2003; Hilditch et al. 2003a; Fellowes et al. 1999).

Nurse-led pre-assessment care offers a comprehensive approach to preparation of the patient for day surgery with the inclusion of: complete history; physical examination; laboratory testing; ECG in determining patient suitability for day surgery; identification of special, cultural and home support requirements; written and verbal information about their procedure (Jeménez et al. 2006). Pre-assessment is considered to be a critical requirement for successful and safe day surgery (NHS Modernisation Agency 2002). Considerable evidence also supports the benefit of nurse-led pre-assessment in reducing the number of DNAs (Did Not Attend), positively impacting on waiting lists by pre-selecting patients suitability in addition to increased levels of patient satisfaction (Clinch 1997; Clark et al. 1999; Clark et al. 2000; Rai and Pandit 2003; Gilmartin 2007).

In addition to the traditional aspects of nurse-led, day surgery pre-assessment, recent innovations demonstrating best practice include telephone screening questionnaires as an effective intervention for pre-admission care (Pearson et al. 2004; Basu et al. 2001). Telephone screening has proven advantages in reducing the number of patients who fail to attend for day surgery. It makes it possible to ascertain the patient's physical condition on the eve of the operation and allows for the reiteration of instructions and information whilst further enhancing the nurse–patient relationship.

Innovations in the reduction of patient anxiety pre-operatively include the institution of distraction therapies such as music as a positive intervention (Cooke et al. 2005; Lee et al. 2004); Mitchell (2000) found that patient anxiety was an area for considerable development and improvement.

A further innovation in nurse-led day surgery pre-assessment is the development of self-managing day surgery nursing teams (Macdonald and Bodzak 1999). Self-managing day surgery nursing teams combine caring, expanded managerial roles, financial responsibility and clinical nursing services successfully. In a longitudinal study by Macdonald and Bodzak (1999), the self-managing day surgery nursing team demonstrated positive staff morale and excellent quality of care, with increased activity and cost-effectiveness. Surprisingly, this approach has not been widely implemented throughout the specialty of day surgery care, quite possibly as a consequence of ill-defined guidance on recommendations for staffing requirements, which appears to be a feature of day surgery from a nursing perspective (Gilmartin 2007).

Nurse-led pre-assessment has also been identified as an area for advanced nursing roles such as nurse practitioner roles. Wu, Walker and Owen (2007) describe a nurse-led clinic for tonsillectomy, whereby direct referral to a nurse-led pre-assessment clinic is by General Practitioners. The nurse practitioner makes the autonomous clinical decision, within an agreed set of protocols, to determine not just the suitability but the necessity to proceed with a planned tonsillectomy and proceeds to complete the surgical pre-assessment and preparation for each of these patients. In a review of the clinic, the DNA rate demonstrated it to be effective and efficient, with complication rates not significantly different from national trends. Innovative practices and roles such as these are paving the way for revolutionary nursing practice within the sphere of nurse-led day surgery care.

Conclusion

Contemporary day surgery has heralded a new era of healthcare knowledge, skills, practices and approaches. Surgical techniques and technological advances, coupled with developments in anaesthetic approaches, have contributed positively to the increase in cases suitable for day surgery, thus contributing to the expansion of services. To facilitate these growing services, innovative methods of ensuring high quality care are required, including specifically designed day surgery units and specialist nurses services, such as nurse-led admission clinics.

The rapid expansion in day surgery internationally will demand ongoing, rapid development of nursing practice to meet the requirements of patients availing themselves of these new services. More importantly, in meeting these challenges, the nursing profession will be required to examine the very nature of its processes, models of care and developments in clinical nursing practice, in order to deliver nursing care that is holistic yet dynamic and reflective of patients' needs. Further consideration is given to the nursing implications of these developments in subsequent chapters.

References

Audit Commission (1990) *A Short Cut to Better Services, Day Surgery in England and Wales.* HMSO, London.

Audit Commission (1991) *Measuring Quality: The Patient's View of Day Surgery.* NHS occasional papers. HMSO, London.

Audit Commission (2001) *Acute Hospital Portfolio – Review of National Findings: Day Surgery.* HMSO, London.

Australian Day Surgery Council (2004) *Day Surgery in Australia: Report and Recommendations of the Australian Day Surgery Council,* revised edition. Royal Australasian College of Surgeons, Australian and New Zealand College of Anaesthetists and the Australian Society of Anaesthetists. Australian Day Surgery Council, Melbourne.

Bain, J., Kelly, H., Snadden, D., Staines, H. (1999) Day surgery in Scotland: Patient satisfaction and outcomes. *Quality in Healthcare,* 8, 86–91.

Basu, S., Babajee, P., Selvachandran, S., Cade, D. (2001) Impact of questionnaires and telephone screening on attendance for ambulatory surgery. *Annals of the Royal College of Surgery of England,* 83, 329–31.

British Association of Day Surgery (2007) http://www.daysurgeryuk.org/content/History/History-of-Day-Surgery.asp (accessed 29 August 2008).

Bureau of Health Planning and Resources Development of the Health Resources Administration USA (1997) *Final Report: Comparative evaluation of costs, quality and system effects of ambulatory surgery performed in alternative settings.*

Cahill, H., Jackson, I. (1997) *Day Surgery Principles and Nursing Practice.* Bailliere Tindall, London.

Cahill, J., Tilin, T. (1995) *Comparative Audit of Day Surgery in the South West Thames Region.* Kingston District Audit Centre, London.

Calnan, J., Martin, P. (1971) Development and practice of an autonomous minor surgery unit in a general hospital. *British Medical Journal,* Vol. iv, 92.

Clark, K., Voase, R., Fletcher, I.R., Thompson, P.J. (1999) Improving patient throughput for oral day case surgery: The efficacy of a nurse-led pre-admission clinic. *Journal of Ambulatory Surgery,* 7, 101–106.

Clark, K., Voase, R., Fletcher, I., Thompson, P. (2000) Patients' experience of oral day case surgery: Feedback from a nurse-led pre-admission clinic. *Ambulatory Surgery,* 8, 93–96.

Clinch, C. (1997) Nurses achieve quality with pre-assessment clinics. *Journal of Clinical Nursing,* 6, 147–151.

Commission on Health Funding Report (1989) *Report of the Commission on Health Funding.* The Stationery Office, Dublin, 1989.

Cooke, M., Chaboyer, W., Schulter, P., Hiratos, M. (2005) The effect of music on preoperative anxiety in day surgery. *Journal of Advanced Nursing,* 52 (1), 47–55.

DeLathouwer, C., Poullier, J.P. (1998) Ambulatory Surgery in 1994–95: The state of art in 29 OECD countries. *Ambulatory Surgery*, 6, 43–55.

Department of Health (2002) *Day Surgery Operational Guide: Waiting, Booking and Choice.* HMSO, London.

Department of Health and Children (1994) *Shaping a Healthier Future: A Strategy for Effective Healthcare in the 1990s.* The Stationery Office, Dublin.

Department of Health and Children (1998) *Executive Summary Report of the Review Group on the Waiting List Initiative.* The Stationery Office, Dublin.

Department of Health and Children (2001a) *Value for Money Audit of the Irish Health System: Executive Summary.* Deloitte & Touche, Dublin.

Department of Health and Children (2001b) *Quality and Fairness: A Health System for You.* The Stationery Office, Dublin.

Department of Health and Children (2002) *Acute Hospital Bed Capacity: A National Review.* The Stationery Office, Dublin.

Department of Health and Children (2003) *The Health Service Reform Programme.* The Stationery Office, Dublin.

Department of Health and Children (2004) *The Modernisation of the National Casemix Programme in Ireland.* The Stationery Office, Dublin.

Department of Health and Children (2005) *Health Statistics 2005.* The Stationery Office, Dublin.

Dooley, W.C. (2002) Ambulatory mastectomy. *The American Journal of Surgery*, 184, 545–9.

Dunn, D. (1998) Pre-operative assessment criteria and patient teaching for ambulatory surgery patients. *Journal of Perianesthesia Nursing*, 13 (5), 274–91.

Epstein, B.S. (2005) Exploring the world of ambulatory surgery. *Journal of Ambulatory Surgery*, 12, 1–5.

Farquharson, E.L. (1955) Early ambulation with special reference to herniorraphy as an outpatient procedure. *Lancet*, Vol. ii, 517–19.

Fellowes, H., Abbott, D., Barton, K., Burgess, L., Clare, A., Lucas, B. (1999) *Orthopaedic Pre-admission Assessment Clinics.* Royal College of Nursing, London.

Gan, T.J., Sloan, F., Dear, G.D.L., El-Moalem, H.E., Lubarsky, D.A. (2001) How much are patients willing to pay to avoid post-operative nausea and vomiting? *Anaesthesia and Analgesia*, 92, 393–400.

Gilmartin, J. (2004) Day surgery: Patients' perceptions of a nurse-led preadmission clinic. *Journal of Clinical Nursing*, 13, 243–50.

Gilmartin, J. (2007) The nurse's role in day surgery: A literature review. *International Nursing Review*, 54 (2), 183–90.

Healthcare Commission (2005) *Acute Hospital Portfolio Review – Inspecting Informing Improving: Day Surgery.*

International Association of Ambulatory Surgery (2003) *World Wide Day Surgery Activity.* IAAS.

Hilditch, W.G., Asbury, A.J., Crawford, J.M. (2003a) Pre-operative screening: Criteria for referring to anaesthetists. *Anaesthesia*, 58 (2), 117–24.

Hilditch, W.G., Asbury, A.J., Jack, E., McGrane, S. (2003b) Validation of a pre-anaesthetic screening questionnaire. *Anaesthesia*, 58 (9), 874–7.

International Association of Ambulatory Surgery (2003) *Ambulatory (Day) Surgery. Suggested International Terminology and Definitions.* http://iaas-med.com/modules/content/Acr977.tmp.pdf (accessed 24 August 2008).

Jenkins, K., Grady, D., Wong, J., Correa, R., Armanious, S., Chung, F. (2001) Postoperative recovery: Day surgery patients' preferences. *British Journal of Anaesthesia*, 86, 272–4.

Jiménez, A., Artigas, C., Elia, M., Casamayor, J.A., Gracia, M., Martinez, M. (2006) Cancellations in ambulatory day surgery: Ten years' observational study. *Journal of Ambulatory Surgery*, 12, 119–23.

Lee, D., Henderson, A., Shum, D. (2004). The effects of music on preprocedure anxiety in Hong Kong Chinese day patients. *Journal of Clinical Nursing*, 13, 297–303.

Macdonald, M., Bodzak, W. (1999) The performance of a self-managing day surgery nurse team. *Journal of Advanced Nursing*, 29, 859–68.

Mitchell, M.J. (2000) Psychological preparation for patients undergoing day surgery. *International Journal of Nursing Studies*, 8 (1), 19–29.

National Health Service Modernisation Agency (2004) *Ten High Impact Changes.* HMSO, London.

National Health Service Modernisation Agency (2002) *Operating Theatre and Pre-operative Assessment Programme.* HMSO, London.

National Health Service Value For Money Unit. (1989) Bevan Report. *A Study of the Management and Utilisation of Operating Departments.* (Bevan Report). HMSO, London.

National Health Service Value For Money Unit. (1991) *Day Surgery: Making it Happen.* HMSO, London.

National Health Service Management Executive (1993) *Day Surgery: Report by the Day Surgery Task Force.* NHS Management Executive, Department of Health, London.

Nicoll, J.H. (1909) The surgery of infancy. *British Medical Journal*, 18, 753–55.

Nightingale, F. (1914) *Notes on Nursing.* Harrison & Son, London.

Ormrod, G., Casey, D. (2004) The educational preparation of nursing staff undertaking pre-assessment of surgical patients: a discussion of the issues. *Nurse Education Today*, 24 (4), 269–76.

Palumbo, L.T., Paul, R.E., Emery, F.B. (1952) Results of primary inguinal hernioplasty. *Archives of Surgery*, Vol. 64, 384–94.

Pearson, A., Richardson, M., Cairns, M. (2004) 'Best practice' in day surgery units: A review of the evidence. *Journal of Ambulatory Surgery*, 11, 49–54.

Rai, M.R., Pandit, J.J. (2003) Day of surgery cancellations after a nurse-led pre-assessment in an elective surgical centre: The first 2 years. *Anaesthesia*, 58 (7), 692–9.

Royal College of Surgeons (1985) *Report of the Working Party on Guidelines for Day Case Surgery.* Royal College of Surgeons, London.

Royal College of Surgeons (1992) *Guidelines for Day Case Surgery.* Royal College of Surgeons, London.

Scott, N.B., Hodson, M. (1997) Public perceptions of post-operative pain and its relief. *Anaesthesia*, 52, 438–42.

Seibert, J.H., Brien, J.S., Maaske, B.L., Kochura, K., Feldt, K., Fader, L., Race, K. E.H. (1999) Assessing patient satisfaction across the continuum of ambulatory care:

A revalidation and validation of care specific surveys. *Journal of Ambulatory Care Management*, 22 (2), 9–26.

Waters, R.M. (1919) The down-town anesthesia clinic. *American Journal of Surgery*, 33 (suppl.), 71–73.

Wu, K., Walker, E., Owen, G. (2007) Nurse-led 'one-stop' clinic for elective tonsillectomy referrals. *Journal of Laryngology and Otology*, 1, 4.

Yeng, Y.P., Cheung, F.L., Chun, A.Y.W. (2002) Survey on post-operative pain control in ambulatory surgery in Hong Kong Chinese. *Journal of Ambulatory Surgery*, 10, 21–24.

Models of Care

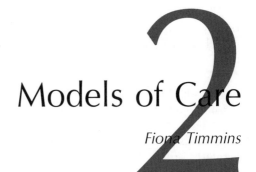

Fiona Timmins

Introduction

Both nursing students and qualified nurses will be very familiar with the term 'nursing models'. There has been much time and energy devoted over the past 30 years to both development and discussion of nursing models and their potential contribution to nursing. Conceptual models of nursing were developed to guide the assessment, planning, intervention and evaluation of nursing care. Primarily aimed at changing nurses' way of thinking away from a medical approach towards care towards a more holistic model of care that considers the person, they also have served to support a movement towards the professionalisation of nursing (Timmins 2005). Most nurses are familiar with conceptual model use in practice. The Roper, Logan, Tierney conceptual model (RLT) (Roper et al. 1980, 1985, 1990, 1996) is an example of a commonly used conceptual model of nursing: it underpins much assessment and care planning documentation across the UK and Ireland; other models are less well known in the practice domain.

Despite their relative popularity, conceptual models of nursing have undergone limited testing in terms of their ability to make a difference to patient outcome (Tierney 1998; Taylor et al. 2000) and this fact, together with their association with increased paper work, compound an apathy that oft-times exists within the profession towards their use. This is disappointing, given the relative youth of many of the conceptual models, for without comprehensive testing in practice they remain at a neophyte developmental stage (Timmins 2005).

This neophyte developmental stage of conceptual models is certainly reflected in day surgery settings, for which no one particular conceptual model of nursing has been advocated. There is also little reported use of these models in day surgery within the literature. However, they are recommended for use in day surgery to promote holistic care (Hodge 1999). A further support for their use is patient-reported experience in the area. Given the high volume of patients using this service and the repetitiveness of the procedures, patients can sometimes feel that that they are not recognised as individuals but rather as a condition while receiving care (Costa 2001). Similarly, some studies report patient dissatisfaction due to with lack of information received and poor discharge planning (Otte 1996; Mitchell 1997; James 2000). These factors, together with the challenge of potential erosion to modern nursing through the taking on of tasks which were previously within the medical domain (Thompson 2002), encourage nurses to seek out frameworks for care delivery that essentially emanate from the profession itself and are ultimately patient-centred. It is suggested that nurses base their practice upon nursing theory (Alligood and Marriner-Tomey 2002a; Fawcett 1999) within the complexity of modern day surgery, providing a more seamless, holistic and integrated approach; this may require a conceptual model of nursing that could comprehensively provide for patient care, which a closer examination of conceptual models of nursing may serve to inform.

Outline of conceptual models of nursing care

Hodge (1999) suggests that all conceptual models are concerned with the individual, health, nursing and the environment or society, and that each theorist's view on these aspects of living are influenced by their particular philosophy. This is a very easy way to understand the traditional abstract presentation by Fawcett (1995) of the metaparadigm, defined as global concepts that identify the phenomena that are of interest to any discipline. This delineation of a metaparadigm relates to a conceptual understanding of the hierarchy of nursing knowledge: firstly there is a metaparadigm; secondly a philosophy; thirdly theory; and fourthly a conceptual model of nursing. It is the conceptual models that practicing nurses are most familiar with, and their use provides for a logical, systematic approach, with particular emphasis on assessment, planning, implementing and evaluation of care, one that is less reliant on tradition and personal nurse preference. Applying this systematic approach to nursing care has particular resonance in day surgery settings. In particular, accurate patient assessment, which is required to determine suitable patients and prepare them for surgery to prevent unnecessary delays, cancellations and disruption to patients. Increasingly nurses in day surgery settings are involved in pre-admission assessment of patients to address some of these issues and this will be discussed in Chapter 3. This congruence between nursing practices in day surgery and a systematic approach to nursing care suggests that conceptual model use in this area may be useful.

Selection and use of a conceptual model of nursing has, in the past, often been a matter for the individual hospital concerned (Hodge 1999). In general, if conceptual models are used in a hospital setting, one model is used or adapted for use across all health care settings. There are obvious advantages to this, as having several models in operation could prove difficult to manage, but disadvantages also arise when attempts are made to ensure that one model fits all, if appropriate modifications are not made. This is particularly so in day surgery; it can be quite disadvantageous if the accepted hospital conceptual model based documentation (CMBD) is lengthy, as might be required in areas with a lower patient turnover. It is reassuring to know that there is a move towards careful and thoughtful selection of conceptual models of nursing within specific areas (Timmins 2005), which means that the hospital's approach to CMBD can be suitably adapted to the day surgery unit. Even if a conceptual model is in use in the day surgery area, a thorough re-examination of its usefulness and contribution can prove a useful exercise, perhaps through local audit. By identifying areas that may require improvement, successful adaptation may increase their usefulness.

Selection of a conceptual model of nursing entails liaison with key members of staff to identify the philosophy of the unit and matching the philosophy to the most appropriate model (Timmins 2005). An innovative approach that invites ownership from nursing staff is beneficial to successful adaptation and there are several examples of this in the literature (McClune and Franklin 1987; Sutcliffe 1994; Graeme 2000). Selection of a conceptual model can also follow with *suitable* adaptation of the model to the area. Fawcett (1995) recommends an eight-stage, phased approach to conceptual model selection, firstly articulating a collective vision and in the second phase getting together a dedicated group of nurses to determine whether implementation is feasible. If the use of conceptual models appears feasible, a third phase begins, whereby a specific planning group is developed to oversee the project. In phase four documents from the area are reviewed, including the mission statement and philosophy (Fawcett 1995). In the fifth phase a conceptual model is chosen by staff, having compared various conceptual models to the unit's beliefs and values. Education of nursing staff is essential and forms the sixth phase. Phase seven, a pilot introduction of the model, is followed by the eighth and final phase of widespread adoption. From a practical perspective, Sutcliffe (1994) outlines a good working example of staff coming together to develop a unit philosophy and subsequently using this to aid selection of a model of nursing. During a previous audit it appeared that the model in use was not achieving its overall aims, as nurses were using their own personal approaches to care, which caused confusion for nursing students and new staff. The staff subsequently used and adapted the RLT conceptual model (Roper et al. 1980, 1985, 1990, 1996), renamed the Mead Model (Sutcliffe 1994).

Ensuring that a conceptual model is congruent with the unit philosophy or the values held by the nurses is crucial to decision-making when considering model usage (Alligood and Marriner-Tomey 2002b). This matching of philosophies and beliefs is an approach that is also suggested for model selection day surgery settings (Hodge 1999). By outlining the core elements of day surgery nursing, Hodge (1999) suggests that these could be used to determine the suitability of choice of conceptual model (Box 2.1).

One difficulty that can arise in the practice setting is ambivalence towards conceptual model use (Murphy et al. 2000). Conceptual model use, while providing detailed documentation to support assessing, planning, implementing and evaluating nursing care, has become synonymous with documentation. Nurses spending long periods completing this documentation can feel frustration that it may take away from direct patient care (Mason 1999). It is also found that documentation of nursing care is not taken to completion, for example, the evaluative component may be missing (Murphy et al. 2000). Furthermore, this compartmentalising of conceptual models within documentation served to develop a somewhat lip service approach (Mason and Chandley 1992; Hyde et al. 2006). This means that while many clinical areas profess to use conceptual models, they may be little more than a paper exercise (Griffiths 1998). Studies indicate that nurses continue to operate from within their own personal or organisational frameworks; these are not necessarily linked to the underpinning philosophy or orientation of

---

Box 2.1   *The core elements of day surgery nursing* (Hodge 1999)

■ **Man:** a unique biosocial complex human being who has individual needs of a spiritual, physical, social and psychological nature, which when addressed will:
  1. promote safe preparation for surgery and care in the unit and
  2. promote reintegration to role and society following discharge from the unit
■ **Nursing:** achieved through partnership and interaction using a systematic approach to care to promote a safe and speedy return to role and society by the patient; the nurse is a specialist in the area of day surgery and an expert communicator and educator.
■ **Environment:** provides a feeling of safety, reassurance, comfort and expertise.
■ **Health:** the integration and re-integration following surgery to the individual's usual role in society.

the conceptual model in use (Mason and Chandley 1992; Griffiths, 1998; Murphy et al. 2000; Treacy and Hyde 2003). The process of selection and subsequent buying into a conceptual model of nursing is vital: otherwise, conceptual model use becomes an exercise that is burdensome on staff and has little impact on overall quality of care. In particular, excessive documentation associated with assessing, planning, implementing and evaluating care in day surgery settings would be not only burdensome but almost impossible to fully complete in a timely fashion, thus rendering the exercise of limited use. Selection of an appropriate conceptual model of nursing requires an examination of how the model can be succinctly applied to day care.

In relation to suggesting a conceptual model for use in day surgery, Hodge (1999) does not proffer any answers. Acknowledging that there are 'similarities' between several conceptual models and the approach required in day surgery, she suggests that 'no one established framework has the complete answer' (Hodge 1999:147). Given the short stay of patients in day surgery settings, a conceptual model of nursing approach that is not overly cumbersome is recommended. Hodge (1999: 150) devised a framework for care in day-care surgery, outlining several 'care phases': pre-admission assessment (suitability for day surgery); arrival and preparation; procedure; recovery; discharge; and immediate and long-term follow up.

Interestingly, Hodge (1999) does not suggest any similarities between the RLT model (Roper et al. 1980, 1985, 1990, 1996) and core elements of day surgery nursing, although Orem's Self-Care Deficit Nursing Theory (SCDNT) (Orem 1971, 1980, 1985, 1995, 2001) is suggested. Given the popularity in practice of the former and the relatively widespread testing associated with the latter (Berbiglia 2002), these two conceptual models will now be briefly discussed to examine their potential contribution to day surgery nursing. Reference to seminal texts will be necessary to develop a deeper understanding of the topic under consideration.

The Roper, Logan and Tierney model

Developed in UK (Edinburgh), the RLT model (Roper et al. 1980, 1985, 1990, 1996) identifies five factors associated with the condition of living:

- The need to perform Activities of Living
- The nature of a persons lifespan
- The presence of a dependence/independence continuum
- Factors that can influence a persons ability to perform Activities of Living
- A persons' individuality.

These factors explain, from the authors' perspective, the human condition. We all need to perform certain activities in order to live – Roper et al.

Box 2.2 *Activities of Living* *(Roper et al. 1980, 1985, 1990, 1996)*

Maintaining a safe environment
Communicating
Breathing
Eating and drinking
Eliminating
Personal cleansing and dressing
Controlling body temperature
Working and playing
Mobilising
Sleeping
Expressing sexuality
Dying

(1980, 1985, 1990, and 1996) identify 12 of these (Box 2.2) – and we are all influenced by where we are in terms of our own lifespan. Individual activities and needs vary depending upon one's age, and also when the dependence/independence continuum is considered. A young baby is considered dependent and an adult independent, but there are a variety of levels in between. Of course not all adults are fully independent. There are many factors that affect a person's ability to perform Activities of Living and many of these necessitate nursing care. A person who has a bunion (Hallux Valgus), for example, may have difficulty walking and thus require day surgery and associated nursing and medical care (Kitson 2007).

Individuality in living is probably where the RLT model has made its biggest contribution (Tierney 1998), assisting nurses to move away from what Fawcett (1999) terms 'romance' with the medical profession, manifested by preoccupation with the medical approach, which isn't always appropriate for nurses or patients. Considering the patient's individuality as Roper et al. (1980, 1985, 1990, 1996) have done, provides for a more meaningful and personalised approach to patient care. Within day surgery settings, patients are often not satisfied with an approach that they perceive not to be individualised, hence the benefits of using this model are immediately obvious. There is a tendency in specialised areas like day surgery, where there is a high throughput of patients with similar conditions all requiring treatment under intense time pressures, for a routine approach to care to occur that can become depersonalised. While routines are obviously important, it is also important for nurses to retain an individual, patient-centered focus, whether or not conceptual models are used.

Using the nursing process (assess, plan, implement and evaluate) within the RLT framework provides the nurse with an opportunity to interview the patient and their family and document the patients' problems or needs related to each particular activity. It has already been identified that paper-work associated with conceptual model use is very cumbersome for practising nurses, and with the short turnaround times associated with patient care in day surgery settings, the level of documentation required could prove even more onerous and perhaps even self-limiting. Furthermore, an oft-cited difficulty with use of the model is the appropriateness of *all* activities to each area. Should a nurse in day surgery require to know about a patient's expression of their sexuality? The potential non-requirement of some areas may need consideration during potential adaptation. Consideration of the RLT model for particular day surgery units may be carried out using the processes mentioned later in this chapter. A further conceptual model is briefly considered to help to inform local choices. Orem's conceptual model will now be described.

Orem's self-care deficit theory of nursing

Orem's *Self-Care Deficit Nursing Theory* (SCDNT) (Orem 1971, 1980, 1985, 1995, 2001) comprises firstly a Self-Care Deficit Theory of Nursing (SCDNT) that underpins the models developed. This represents a theory of what nursing is and should be and is a general guide to practice. The SCDNT theory suggests that:

- People require continuous input from both themselves and their environment in order to function.
- There is a agency associated with being human, represented by an ability to act deliberately that motivates and drives needs-based self-care and that of others.
- Agency is something that develops gradually in people, over time, and allows independence with regard to personal actions and decisions.
- Humans experience limitations on their own self-care and that of others.

Within the SCDNT theory there are three intertwining theories of self-care, self-care deficit and nursing systems (Orem 2001). These explain the human condition. Self-care is learned and permits people to deliberately care for themselves and others. Self-care deficit explains why people may require nursing care, whereby they are unable to independently perform self-care or care of others. People require nursing care if their need for care exceeds their own capacity to attend to these needs, which can be temporary or permanent. In the day surgery setting this deficit relationship is usually temporary. The theory of nursing systems explains that nursing is a deliberate human action by nurses arising from their *nursing agency* to provide care to people with self-care deficits. The nurses' role within this theory is very much that of a helper (Orem 2001):

- Acting for or doing for another
- Guiding and directing
- Providing physical or psychological support
- Providing and maintaining an environment that supports Personal development
- Teaching.

Within this nursing system, nursing care can be described as either *wholly compensatory* (doing for the patient), *partly compensatory* (helping the patient to do for himself or herself), or *supportive-educative* (helping the patient learn to do for himself or herself).

Orem (2001) also describes self-care requisites that exist or potentially exist within the human condition. These are universal self-care requisites, developmental self-care requisites and health deviation self-care requisites. Universal self-care requisites are eight universally required goals that are met through self-care or dependent care to maintain adequate functioning and human development:

- Maintaining sufficient intake or air, water and food and elimination processes
- Maintaining a balance between activity/rest and solitude/social interaction
- Preventing hazards to human life
- Promotion of human functioning and development within social groups.

Developmental self-care requisites pertain to processes of life and maturation and prevent situations that could adversely affect these processes. Health deviation self-care requisites are self-care requisites that exist for persons who are ill, injured, disabled or undergoing medical diagnosis and/ or treatment.

Using the nursing process (assess, plan, implement and evaluate) within Orem's framework also provides the nurse with an opportunity to interview the patient and their family and document the patients' self-care deficits related to each particular activity. Assessment involves an estimation of the therapeutic self-care demand through analysis of therapeutic self-care requisites in three distinct domains: universal, health deviation, and developmental. Planning involves identification of self-care requisites and the process for meeting these. Intervention involves nursing agency to meet patients' therapeutic self-care demands and to promote patients' self-care agency (Orem 2001).

The teaching role identified within this conceptual model (Orem 2001) has important implications for day surgery which will be further developed in Chapter 4. Patients report being inadequately prepared for day surgery from an information perspective and thus being under-prepared for their procedure (Otte 1996). As communication- and information-giving is identified as having a central role in day surgery, a conceptual model of nursing that harnesses communication as a central tenet is now described (Peplau 1952, 1991).

Peplau's conceptual frame of reference for psychodynamic nursing

You may not necessarily associate Peplau's (1952, 1991) work with traditional conceptual models of nursing, as it enjoys a close association with informing communication skills for nurses because of its emphasis on developing a relationship between nurse and patient. Referred to in most contemporary nursing communication texts, Peplau's (1952, 1991) Conceptual Frame of Reference for Psychodynamic Nursing holds that nursing is concerned with patient growth and development sustained through relationship with the nurse. It is commonly used as a framework upon which to base interventions in psychiatric nursing, and indeed Barker (2001) has further developed and built upon its inherent concepts to develop an appropriate model for care within mental health settings.

Peplau (1952, 1991) suggests that the nurse–patient relationship, or partnership, develops in distinct phases. These phases are admission, intervention, recovery and discharge. During each of these phases, the nurse may be involved in orientation, identification, exploitation or resolution, or a mixture of these. Peplau (1952, 1991) outlines specific nursing actions during these phases, for example during orientation (related to admission, intervention, recovery or discharge) the nurse may act as a resource person, a listener or technical expert. The nurse and patient work together to identify patient needs. Identification refers to the development of a nurse–patient relationship, whereby the patient strongly identifies with the nurse caring for them. This professional relationship aids recovery. Once identification takes place, the patient is encouraged to *exploit*, that is to say, make full use of the services available, and the nurse can facilitate this. The patient feels aware and confident to utilise the resources available in the health-care context. Once goals have been achieved, resolution occurs and new goals are formed for discharge. Peplau (1952, 1991) also identifies other nursing roles such as teacher. The nurse–patient relationship is a central tenet within this approach.

Although it may be argued that day surgery settings allow little time to develop relationships between nurse and client (Otte1996), ironically the final outcome of the experience depends upon good advice and preparation for discharge that the patient receives from the nurse (Howard-Harwood 1997). Increasingly there is an emphasis within health upon not only the nurse–patient relationship but also on becoming patient-centred (McCabe and Timmins 2004). There are also calls to improve nurses' communication skills – in some day surgery settings, patients report deficits in these (Rogan Foy and Timmins 2004). Patients sometimes report a breakdown in communication during their day surgery experience (Otte 1996). These factors together with the relative simplicity of the use of Peplau's (1952, 1991) model make it worthy of consideration within day surgery settings. The need for good communication within day surgery settings (further developed in Chapter 7), makes this a useful model for consideration for use in day surgery.

While all three conceptual models explored within this chapter contain specific elements that may be useful to practising nurses in day surgery settings, in order to determine what contribution a conceptual model could potentially make to a particular area of nursing it is important to evaluate this contribution prior to adoption.

Evaluation of the contribution of conceptual models of nursing to day surgery practice

In the past, conceptual models were often adopted uncritically by nurses in practice, with resultant apathy regarding use when they didn't work well. Critical appraisal is an essential step in the process of implementation of conceptual model based practice. Use of systematic frameworks to guide this process is a recurring theme in the literature, with most theoretical texts offering advice in this area.

Cormack and Reynolds (1992) outlined one such framework for evaluating the clinical and practical utility of models used by nurses. They suggested that nurses should evaluate the possible contribution of the model to practice, before selecting it for use. They presented a set of criteria that nurses can use to evaluate a model in order to establish its value in the clinical setting. These criteria are addressed by asking a series of questions about the conceptual model in question (Cormack and Reynolds 1992).

Is the conceptual model:

- Clearly understood by nurses?
- An approach that is specific to nurses and nursing?
- Based on tested and accepted theory?
- Valid and reliable?
- Geographically portable?
- Capable of assisting with the identification of the range of human responses to actual or potential health problems?

Does the conceptual model:

- Provide an explanation for common human responses to health problems experienced by individuals?
- Enable nurses to identify nursing interventions?
- Specify the desired outcome of nursing interventions?
- Comply with accepted ethical standards in nursing?
- Is the conceptual model clearly delineated?

Many writers express the difficulty nurses experience with the understanding of conceptual models and Cormack and Reynolds (1992) suggest that the model should be easy to understand. They suggest that if the average nurse doesn't actually understand it, then the model will be of limited value in practice. The RLT model (Roper et al. 1980, 1985, 1990, 1996), which was used extensively in Europe in the 1980s and 1990s, was noted to be easily understood (Marriner-Tomey 2000) – one reason, perhaps, for its relative popularity.

Cormack and Reynolds (1992) also state that the scope of the model should be clearly delineated. It should also be clear whether or not the model is suitable to day surgery and could potentially meet the needs of the patient group. Most conceptual models purport to have generic application and do not explicitly recommend specific alterations for use in particular settings. However, examination of the theoretical underpinnings of the model, including its definition of nursing, the environment, health and the individual, should assist with outlining its scope.

Cormack and Reynolds (1992) further suggest that a conceptual model should inform nurses in a way that is uniquely nursing orientated. Cormack and Reynolds (1992) also state that a model should provide information about its reliability and validity. This would suggest that a certain level of testing has taken place. Validity relates to whether a model is capable of doing what it professes to do, whereas reliability relates to the ability of the model to produce similar results in similar situations. Finding information on this particular requirement of the author could prove challenging; due to limited testing in practice, this type of information is not always readily available or provided specifically in the relevant core texts.

Cormack and Reynolds (1992) regard geographical portability as a serious issue. They suggest that there has been a trend for models originating in the USA to be applied globally with little specific revision for culturally different nursing situations and that consideration needs to be given to the transferability of both inherent concepts and language to ascertain the model's potential usefulness in the particular setting. Evers (2002) further suggests that a difficulty with language transfer with model use has contributed to a stifling of nursing theory development in Europe. This point is also supported by Shamsudin (2002), who used grounded theory to adapt a conceptual model of nursing to Malyasian nursing practice.

Cormack and Reynolds (1992) also propose that a model should help a nurse to identify patient's problems, provide an explanation for human responses, enable nurses to identify nursing intervention and specify the potential outcome of care. The model should also allow nurses to utilise it within the particular restrictions and responsibilities of their practice domain. For nurses working in day surgery, this would imply that it could be suited to guide care for short-term patient stay. The model ought also to be compliant with ethical principles. To this extent, it should serve to do good and not the opposite.

Using these latter questions to examine the potential benefits of conceptual model based practice can be helpful to nurses in the day surgery unit. It is often difficult to assess the strengths and weaknesses of conceptual models without the assistance of a formalised structure. This suggested framework enables the nurse to make judgements about the conceptual model without over-reliance on anecdotal evidence. It provides an informed and balanced judgement regarding the crucial components of a conceptual model. Consistent with other suggested frameworks identified in the literature, it does not provide guidance such as scoring system to interpret responses; rather, it leaves interpretation open to the user. While this approach may be criticised for lack of direction, it does allow judgement regarding the importance of each item to be worked out at local level.

Evaluation of the contribution of conceptual models of nursing, if in use, to day surgery practice, can be also achieved through quality improvement mechanisms available, such as audit (Hodge 1999). Standards around the use of conceptual models may be developed locally by the team and then the extent to which the required standards are achieved can be measured through a locally developed audit tool. This could seek to ascertain, for example, whether evaluation of care took place. Conceptual models of nursing have not been traditionally associated with standard development, as many of them preceded the era of quality concern. Their primary concern was to articulate and guide a unique approach to nursing care rather than provide for its measurement.

Conceptual model based nursing care intends to achieve a positive changes in both the thinking and practice of nurses. They aim to distance nursing from unnecessary rituals and routines and endeavour to provide frameworks for holistic evidence-based care that is wholly patient-centred. Conceptual model use can serve to strengthen the philosophy of care in particular units and choosing a particular model for day surgery requires careful thought and preparation. It must be said however that the practical benefits to patient care from conceptual model use have received very little scrutiny from a research perspective. Therefore at the outset the benefits are not entirely clear. Furthermore, from reported experiences in the literature, they are undoubtedly synonymous with paperwork and lip-service.

Other ways of conceptualising or delivering nursing care are currently in use. Popular among these is the care pathway. Care pathways provide ability to deliver agreed multidisciplinary care and are proven to reduce costs and increase quality. Thus they hold advantages over the more traditional conceptual models of nursing. However, there is a tendency towards a medical and almost depersonalised approach with their use, which goes against the individualisation and holism that have been professed advantages of conceptual model use by nurses over the decades. Although there is little reported use of care pathways in day surgery in the literature, care pathways have had strong association with positive effects on quality of care (Renholm et al. 2002).

Background and development of care pathways

It is possible that the challenges associated with conceptual model use require 'a reinvention of the nursing care plan . . . without the constraint of a nursing model as the necessary foundation' (Mason 1999: 387). An innovative method of formulating plans of care, termed care pathways, originated in the USA, driven in part by the competitive market of private health care. Embraced as quality measurement initiative that is complicit with the clinical governance agenda, there has been widespread interest and use of care pathways over the past ten years in the UK. The Department of Health supports and endorses their use (Department of Health 1998 a,b).

Although presented as an alternative to conceptual model-based care, their conjoint use is suggested (Pearson et al. 2001). One difficulty associated with the widespread implementation of care pathways is the potential for erosion of conceptual model based care and perhaps even erosion of the very foundations of nursing (Mason 1999). In some instances the concerns are unfounded, as in the development of cardiac care pathways at St Mary's Hospital in Paddington, London. Staff were concerned that the pathways would replace individualised, holistic and nursing process based care but their concerns proved unfounded; the implementation was deemed a success and a great improvement to care in terms of communication, quality and cost, by nursing staff (Stead and Huckle 1997).

What is a care pathway?

There are several terms in use that are associated with care pathway such as integrated care pathways, clinical pathways, and critical pathways, although their use and application has subtle differences (Johnson 1997a). The National Pathway Association (NPA) suggests that a care pathway 'determines locally agreed, multidisciplinary practice based on guidelines and evidence where available, for a specific patient or client group. It forms all or part of the clinical record, documents the care given and facilitates the evaluation of outcomes' (Riley 1998).

Put simply, a care pathway is a specific outline of comprehensive care (rather than specific elements of care) to be provided to a patient group, developed upon consultation and agreement within a range of relevant disciplines. It provides for an evidence-based path of care for a particular patient condition. Although this sometimes includes research, evidence pathways usually reflects consensus-based care rather than evidenced-based care (Holt et al. 1996). They are best suited to commonly performed, straightforward procedures and are usually associated with surgical interventions or medical investigations (Holt et al. 1996), thus making them ideally suited for use within day surgery settings. They are primarily used within hospitals and their use does not usually extend beyond discharge (Holt et al. 1996).

The care pathway outlines the usual assessment, interventions and treatment and ultimate outcome expected from a range of health professionals when a patient presents with the relevant condition. By outlining the range of experiences a patient is expected to have on their journey, these can be signed off, upon patient discharge, as complete. This clearly acts as a guide to new and junior staff to ensure that care interventions are not forgotten; more importantly, it can be easily observed whether or not specific interventions took place. In a sense this is a tick-box approach to care but it allows measurement of outcomes, the jewel in the crown of care pathways. Some believe that pathways represent a retrograde step in nursing practice, because the standardised care that pathways provide, while improving overall quality of care, potentially reduce the person-centred approach. However strength of pathway use lies in the focus on evaluation of the process. The pathway usually contains key elements of care and treatment for a particular condition or disease. Its documentation often takes the form of a grid, indicating a timescale at the top (days or hours) and a vertical list of interventions. Deviations that occur with the use of the plan in practice are called 'variances'. Through analysis of the level and number of variances with a particular condition, monitoring of current practice can take place (Johnson 1997b). These data can then be used to update and improve clinical practices by incorporating any new changes within the overall pathway template, thus completing the audit cycle (Kitchiner et al. 1996, Campbell et al. 1998). The pathway becomes a dynamic tool that is continually being refined.

It is important to note that, unlike conceptual models of nursing, care pathways are multidisciplinary and their use is also supported within other health care occupations (Johnson 1997b). Joint use among disciplines encourages an increased partnership approach to care and prevents care fragmentation. Care pathways are frequently used among NHS Trust Hospitals in the UK, mostly in the areas of orthopaedic surgery and cardiac nursing (Riley 1998). They are often used as the basis of multidisciplinary documentation, clinical guidelines and quality standards (Riley 1998; De Luc 2000).

There are several useful resources available to staff interested in their use. The National Day Surgery Association (UK) expands the earlier definition of care pathway and use the term *integrated* care pathway to describe an outline of care for one patient group (Fisher and McMillan 2004). This publication outlines the development, implementation and evaluation of integrated care pathways for day surgery and provides for useful reading in the area (Fisher and McMillan 2004). There is also an international journal dedicated to pathways: *Journal of Integrated Care Pathways*, and a UK-based, yearly *integrated care pathway* conference. A National Electronic *Protocols & Care Pathways Specialist Library* (NHS 2008a) also exists as a subcomponent of The NHS National Library for Health (NHS 2008b). This website provides a Care Pathways Database presented from over 200 NHS organisations. There are several examples provided from NHS hospitals related to day surgery including: hand surgery; removal of metal work in the hand/arm; removal of metal work in the leg; wrist surgery; vasectomy; and minor gynaecology. Although these pathways are useful for reference purposes, it is suggested that pathways should either be developed or modified locally to suit particular needs of the specific patient group, rather than using predetermined pathways (Wall and Proyect 1998). Care pathways should be developed collaboratively within the local health care team. There is some discussion within the literature about how this may be done.

Developing care pathways

Wall and Proyect (1998) suggest that establishing and determining a collaborative understanding of terminology related to care pathways is an important first step. This can be assisted by examining existing definitions. Inatavicius and Hausmann (1995) describe methods for development and implementation of pathways. They identify the two essential factors that are necessary for successful implementation as support from a hospital's administration team and resources. They also recommend the appointment of a project manager to lead the development, as commitment of dedicated staff is more likely to yield success.

Multidisciplinary support for project is also important, and once support for the development is established, a steering group may be established to guide the project. They further suggest that the selection of the pathway involves three steps, selection of the target pathway, establishment of the outcome(s) to achieve by using a pathway for the target population, determine aspects of care to include in the pathway (Inatavicius and Hausmann 1995).

Upon review of several day surgery related care pathways included in the Protocols and Care Pathways Specialist Library (NHS 2008a) there is an obvious tendency for the outline of interventions to resemble as straight forward list of medical interventions that need to be done. While this has obvious usefulness in terms of ensuring that nothing gets forgotten, there is a sense that the nursing element of the care is somehow consumed within a medical model of care, albeit a interdisciplinary approach. An examination of the literature in relation to the nurses' role in day surgery may illuminate the way in which local pathways could be developed that could retain the required nursing focus.

Mitchell (2006) highlights that increases in day surgery provision have led to a 'rapid change in surgical healthcare delivery' with a resultant 'shift of emphasis in surgical nursing intervention' and that this has rendered the nursing emphasis almost invisible (Mitchell 2006). Many surgical interventions such as inguinal hernia repair, varicose vein stripping, cataract extraction and cholecystectomy being just a few of the surgical interventions that previously required and are now being provided on a one day basis, closely managed by medical protocols (Mitchell 2006). While the constant evolution of day surgery services represents a challenge to the currently 'multitasking' nurse in these settings Mitchell (2006) is confident that specific aspects of care that fall within the domain of nursing as previously mentioned (pain management, pre-assessment, information giving) together with 'psycho educational' intervention and post operative care will begin to receive increased recognition both locally and nationally. Thus early and innovative inclusion within care pathway development may be forward thinking.

The reduced time spent by day surgery patients in hospital naturally results in a increased emphasis on the medical aspects of care at the possible expense of this traditional psycho-educational intervention. Indeed there is a greater emphasis on self-care (Mitchell 2003). Mitchell (2003) reminds us that over a 40-year period, a substantive body of information has developed attesting to the anxiety-provoking nature of surgery, with specific fears emerging in relation to anaesthetic, the operation and unconsciousness. While nurses traditionally had time to prepare and reassure patients when required, short-stay surgery militates against this. Information provision to day surgery patients is covered in more detail in Chapter 4. At this point, it is sufficient to say that from a care pathway perspective, Mitchell (2000) suggests that nurses working in day surgery have a distinct role with regard to anxiety management and proposes an 'anxiety management care plan' to be used in conjunction with a 'structured programme of information provision'. Comprehensive and sensitive information booklets would form part of this approach (Mitchell 2007).

Indeed, Mitchell (2003) is vociferous in his claim that nurses in day surgery need to be involved in the psychological preparation of patients from pre-admission to post-discharge. Mitchell (2003) describes as 'psycho-educational' elements of care 'a purposeful attempt to provide tangible aspects of care aimed at enhancing an individual's psychological status together with the planned provision of educational material'.

Pain management emerges as a central nursing role within the literature on day surgery. In some cases patients' pain within the day surgery setting was not fully controlled. Susilahti et al. (2004), in a study of 200 Finnish patients, revealed that pain was the most commonly reported problem post-operatively, with 13% believing that analgesia had little effect. Townsend and Cox (2007) discuss pain management for day case orthopaedic surgery emphasising that 'relief of pain is not only a moral and ethical imperative, but there are also physiological reasons why it needs to be treated effectively, particularly with an increasing number of elderly patients now undergoing surgical procedures as a day case.' Strongly associated with the need for readmission, the authors argue that pain assessment is a key nursing role. This involves assessment of the pain (location, nature, pattern, description, intensity, using a numerical rating scale of one to ten, and asking what worsens/lessens pain). They point to the range of pain assessment tools available from the British Pain Society (www.britishpainsociety.org/pub_pain_scales.htm), which also come in a variety of languages. These pain assessment tools, they suggest, should also be provided to patients to use themselves after discharge, as uncontrolled post-operative pain in this period is a recognised problem. They describe a standardised approach to the management of discharge pain, by grouping surgical procedures according to severity and by providing one of three standard pain packs (A,B,C), which provide a varied use of non-steroidal anti-inflammatory medications, paracetamol and codeine based preparations. Education is also part of this process. Similarly, Coll and Ameen (2006), spurred on by doubts expressed 'about the rapid growth of day surgery and its effects on patients' and the dearth of literature in the area, explore the pain experienced by 578 patients following three procedures commonly performed in the day surgery context: hernia surgery; varicose vein excision and laparoscopic sterilisation. Their findings indicated that up to 60% of patients' experienced 'unacceptable' levels of pain on the day of surgery. Uncontrolled pain for many patients continued until at least the third day post-operatively.

Gilmartin and Wright (2007) provide a comprehensive review of the nurse's role in day surgery, indicating that there is an ever increasing impetus to expand and improve day surgery services. Their findings indicate key areas where nursing intervention has been examined and documented within the literature: pre-admission assessment; information giving and anxiety prevention; communication; pain management; wound infection and nausea and vomiting (Gilmartin and Wright 2007). Nausea and vomiting and wound-healing problem are commonly reported following day surgery (Susilahti et al. 2004).These latter areas could form key subsections within the care pathway documentation, around which interventions could be based, and could be adapted to suit each individual care pathway.

An interesting approach to day surgery care emerges from the University Hosptial in Uppsala, Sweden: Bergström (2000) outlines a model of care utilised for day surgical patients, which, although not care pathway based, provides a 'concept of nursing care', whereby four key areas of nursing have been identified. These are information, documentation, care and quality assurance. Care is described as 'individually designed continuity, with follow up postoperative care, telephone call and pain follow up'. An individual care plan is developed for each patient, with patient and family involvement. Clearly, while care pathway development within day surgery settings does not receive much attention within the literature, the nurse's role in this area and nursing priorities (such as: information giving and anxiety prevention; communication; pain management; wound infection and nausea and vomiting) have been identified which could form the basis of care pathway *or* conceptual model based care. This focus on the nursing perspective is particularly important to address some of the criticisms that current care pathways receive in relation to erosion of the specific nursing role. It is useful when considering implementing new approaches to care delivery to observe some working examples and these will now be considered.

Examples of care pathways in current use

Within the Protocols & Care Pathways Specialist Library (NHS 2008a) there are several examples of care pathways submitted by National Health Service (NHS) hospitals (UK). One example from NHS Airedale in Keighley, West Yorkshire is related to ear surgery (NHS 2008a). This comprises two pages of straightforward checklists related to:

- The operation day
- Post-operative period
- Discharge.

These identify the range of expected interventions at each of these stages. There is no provision for variances, although expected outcomes are identified at each stage (Table 2.1).

Table 2.1 Expected outcomes related to ear surgery *(NHS Airdale)*

Phase of Care	Outcomes
The operation day	*Patient demonstrates understanding of:*
	1. Procedure
	2. Discharge plan
	3. Safe and informed patient in theatre
Post-operative period	*Patient demonstrates understanding of:*
	1. Safe recovery from operation and anaesthetic
Discharge	*Patient demonstrates understanding of:*
	1. Plan of discharge attained

The lack of explicit provision to record variances (reasons why interventions were not done, or set goals were not reached) in this example seems to contradict the ethos of the care pathway, as, in order to be relied upon as a quality measurement, records of variances are required. To a certain extent, the pathway is reflective of the medical protocols that predominate in day surgery (Mitchell 2006). This is not to say that such an approach is wrong but rather that the nursing element remains elusive. A detailed record of standard care is, however, provided to nursing staff, which is useful where staff are unfamiliar with the procedures, although, as the pathway concerns all manner of ear surgery, detailed specifics of care are not provided. This documentation may also serve as a prompt to inform patients of their expected journey.

In one other day surgery pathway, Rotherham General Hospital, Trent, UK, provides some space for recording variances. They provide a comprehensive pathway for day surgery to be used for patients attending for minor gynaecology surgery (NHS 2008a). The associated documentation provides for the recording of multidisciplinary care from pre-admission through to discharge, including the theatre experience. To this end they term the pathway an *integrated* care pathway; which as result integrates medical, nursing and other health care intervention. It comprises firstly a pre operative assessment which includes the following:

- demographic details
- hygiene, communication, mobility and nutrition
- proposed mode of transport /accompaniment
- presence of prosthesis
- 'Anxiety/ Fears / Worries?'
- past medical history, serious illnesses, current medications and previous anesthetic history
- required serum blood tests and Electrocardiograph (ECG)
- information leaflets provided (yes or no)
- 'Advised to starve from . . .'

Documentation from the operative day consists of physiological measurements and predication checklist. The documentation later applies to a detailed pre-operative checklist for theatre, and a checklist for use within theatre. Post-operatively, the pathway provides for the observation, measurement and recording of a range of patient physical parameters including:

- Airway
- Breathing
- Consciousness level
- Blood pressure
- Pulse and Respiration rate
- Oxygen saturation
- Intravenous Fluids

- Wound; drains; packs
- Pain (severity rating scale)
- Nausea (severity rating scale)

Some of these latter elements have space to record variance and action taken. It also contains and anaesthetic recording sheet and a checklist to determine fitness for discharge. Medications can also be recorded. This pathway provides a comprehensive guide to all staff working in the day surgery area as to the generic interventions and observations required when caring for patients following minor gynaecological procedures. The pathway comprises ten pages in total, with a series of tables related to each phase of care. There is some element of a nursing focus within the plan, particularly at the pre-admission stage where an assessment of some activities of living is performed. In keeping with Mitchell's (2000, 2003, 2006) concerns about patient anxiety in day surgery settings and the key role that a nurse may play to address this, this element of care is addressed at pre-admission, albeit briefly recorded.

Staff seeking to use either conceptual models of nursing or care pathways commonly request examples of these frameworks in use. The NHS Protocols & Care Pathways Specialist Library (NHS 2008a) is therefore a very useful resource. Airedale NHS Trust provides several examples of care pathways that vary individually in construction. These include:

- Day case – vasectomy
- Day surgery – dental surgery
- Day surgery – hand surgery
- Day surgery – removal of metal work arm
- Day surgery – removal of metal work leg
- Day surgery – wrist surgery

These examples of pathways in use provide a good template for those working in day surgery units that are considering care pathway implementation. Although their approach varies, standardised care for each condition appears to be provided and in accordance with pathway aims there is some provision for brief evaluation of the process, in so far as whether the intervention was done or not. The care pathway documentation comprises eight pages, with distinct tables related to admission, recording of variance and discharge (Table 2.2). The pathway contains essential generic elements of care and treatment for hand surgery, which is in keeping with care pathway development. Its documentation permits detailed recording of variance, which can assist with quality measurement, however a timescale at the top (days or hours) is not provided with the list of interventions, perhaps as the timescale is limited in day surgery to one day. The hand surgery care pathway example from NHS Airedale (NHS 2008a) firstly comprises an *admission day* checklist (Table 2.2). This form (on the left side of Table 2.2) denotes one page of documentation. Similarly the patient outcomes and

Table 2.2 Hand surgery care pathway example from NHS Airedale *(NHS 2008a). Admission checklist, expected outcomes table for recording variances.*

ADMISSION DAY		Date	Variance	Action Taken
MEDICAL				
Medical Assessment				
Operation explained / Mark appropriate wrist				
Consent obtained				
Prescribe all medication				
NURSING				
Nursing Assessment				
R P B/P				
Weight				
Introduce to named nurse				
Provide Op-Fax information				
Explore any anxieties				
Inform location of fire exits				
Assess for self/med	Y / N			
Complete admission book				
Identity bracelet				
Red identity for allergy	Y / N			
Introduce to ward routines				
Provide ward info book				
Check Op site marked				

OUTCOMES (please tick)	
Patient demonstrates understanding of:	
1. Plan of care *achieved ...... not achieved ......*	
2. Fasting Protocol *achieved ...... not achieved ......*	
3. Discharge Date *achieved ...... not achieved ......*	

OUTCOMES (please tick)

Outcome 1	**On Path**	
Patient demonstrates understanding of plan of care	Late	
	Early	
	Relapsed	
	Not Achieved	
	Not Applicable	
Outcome 2	**On Path**	
Patient demonstrates understanding of plan of care	Late	
	Early	
	Relapsed	
	Not Achieved	
	Not Applicable	
Outcome 3	**On Path**	
Patient demonstrates understanding of plan of care	Late	
	Early	
	Relapsed	
	Not Achieved	
	Not Applicable	
Outcome 4	**On Path**	
Patient demonstrates understanding of plan of care	Late	
	Early	
	Relapsed	
	Not Achieved	
	Not Applicable	

table to record variances (on the right) are also afforded one full page each. The care pathway, unlike the integrated approach of Rotherham General Hospital in the last example, focuses solely upon admission and later discharge. The related discharge documentation is outlined in Table 2.3. There is firstly a full page devoted to discharge home, which outlines nursing interventions (on the right hand side of the table). There is space to record whether the four previously described outcomes have been achieved. A list of discharge criteria is also provided as a one page document. Variances from the pathway may be recorded.

Contemporary nursing practice is concerned with delivering high quality care in the context of clinical effectiveness. Patient care ought to be delivered in a patient-centred way in partnership with both patient and family. Day surgery services are associated with a high turnover of patients, and the nurse working in these settings needs to be not only flexible and adaptable but knowledgeable in a wide spectrum of surgical interventions and their subsequent management and care. Recent movements within National Health Service provision suggest the use of care pathways to guide the delivery of patient care. These have specific advantages to care delivery, including the ability to provide for locally developed and agreed standards of care (NCNM 2006). It is also suggested that they permit good communication of protocol and interventions, through clear documentation that can enhance confidence, empowerment and teamwork care (NCNM 2006). Associated documentation is thought to be easy to use, as the majority of recording relates to variances that might occur in care (2006). Most importantly care pathways allow 'clinical analysis of care practices and results through monitoring of progress according to pre-established outcomes, thereby optimising professional accountability and ensuring an opportunity for continuous quality improvement of patient care.' (NCNM 2006;10)

While limited testing of their usefulness in day surgery settings, the inclusion of several examples of day surgery pathways on the NHS Protocols & Care Pathways Specialist Library (NHS 2008a) is a testament to their usefulness in practice. With both local hospital and national policy acceptance and support, they do seem a useful framework not only to direct and guide nursing care, but within which to both operate and measure clinical effectiveness of care. Unlike conceptual model selection, there is limited guidance within the literature to care pathway selection, although the NHS Protocols & Care Pathways Specialist Library (NHS 2008a) provides several interesting links for 'care pathways development'.

It does seem disappointing that conceptual models of nursing, in so far as care pathways are concerned, are very much falling by the wayside in favour of more time sensitive, comprehensive and specific plans of care. Given Gilmartin and Wright's (2007) outline of the role of the nurse in day surgery focusing on the key areas of: pre-admission assessment; information giving and anxiety prevention; communication; pain management; wound infection and nausea and vomiting, and Mitchell's (2000, 2003,

Table 2.3 Hand surgery care pathway example from NHS Airedale *(NHS 2008a). Discharge checklist, expected outcomes table for recording variances.*

DISCHARGE HOME DAY			
NURSING	**Date**	**Variance**	**Action Taken**
Complete discharge plan			
Inform relatives			
Order TTOs			
Obtain TTOs / explain to patient			
Transport			
Give written discharge advice–explain ontent if necessary			
Make appointment follow up clinic in 2 weeks			
Practice Nurse Appointment for			
ROS 7–10 days if BH			
Outcome (please tick)			
Safely discharged home or to an appropriate			
Place of care *achieved* ...... *not achieved*			

Discharge criteria	Yes	No	N/A
Do you have someone responsible at home to care for you?			
Is there going to be a responsible person/relative to collect you?			
Are you ALLERGIC to any food or medicine?			
Have you been given your take home medicines?			
Do you require a sick note from the doctor?			
Have written and verbal advice/instructions been given and understood?			
Have a District/Practice nurse appointment been made?			
Are/is the patients:			
Vital signs stable?			
Alert and orientated?			
Diet and fluids taken and tolerated?			
Pain and nausea controlled?			
Voided urine?			
Pack/drain removed?			
Wound checked?			
Dressing changed/supply given?			
Venflon removed?			
ECG pads removed?			
Time of discharge and with whom/carer at home?			

Outcome 1	**On Path**	
Patient demonstrates understanding of plan of care	Late	
	Early	
	Relapsed	
	Not Achieved	
	Not Applicable	
Outcome 2	**On Path**	
Patient demonstrates understanding of plan of care	Late	
	Early	
	Relapsed	
	Not Achieved	
	Not Applicable	
Outcome 3	**On Path**	
Patient demonstrates understanding of plan of care	Late	
	Early	
	Relapsed	
	Not Achieved	
	Not Applicable	
Outcome 4	**On Path**	
Patient demonstrates understanding of plan of care	Late	
	Early	
	Relapsed	
	Not Achieved	
	Not Applicable	

2006) assertion that day surgery nursing has a vital role to play in both pre-hospital and in-hospital anxiety management, it is likely that specific nursing actions within these key areas could be further expanded within care pathway development. In particular the nurse–patient relationship needs to be emphasised and drawn upon to document the engagement with patients that takes place (or ought to take place). Current trends relate not only to high standards of care delivery, and timely and equal access to treatment: there is also a requirement that patients and their family are 'treated with dignity, respect and empathy at all times'; furthermore, patients and family need to be involved in, and informed about, all decisions made during their journey of care (NHS Quality Improvement Scotland 2005:8). It is questionable the extent to which this element of nursing care is provided for within a care pathway approach. This is not to say that it does not occur but rather that there is often not a direct account given of it, unlike conceptual model based care, which does so either implicitly or explicitly, due to its extrapolation of the metaparadigm. Unfortunately there is always the risk that reducing the patient's hospital experience to a series of tasks may result in a feeling of depersonalisation, as was expressed in Costa's (2001) study. It is of interest to note that, within the many professed benefits of care pathways, improving the patient's experience, from an emotional perspective is not alluded to (NCNM 2006, NHS Quality Improvement Scotland 2005). These tacit expressions of nursing, which are so often present but perhaps not accounted for, could perhaps be better harnessed by incorporating at least some element of conceptual model based care within the day surgery unit. This could, at the very least, comprise a unit philosophy and statement about the conceptual model based care to which it subscribes. The use of a conceptual model of nursing could perhaps revert to the purpose that it once had, before it became over-consumed by paperwork, as a mental representation for nurses of how nursing should be. For example, constituent elements of the RLT model (Roper et al. 1980, 1985, 1990, 1996) could be used to underpin assessment, as in the example from Rotherham General Hospital above. Similarly, Orem's Self-Care Deficit Nursing Theory (SCDNT) (Orem, 1971, 1980, 1985, 1995, 2001) could be used to underpin core beliefs, as self-care is very much a part of contemporary day surgery (Mitchell 2007). Furthermore, given the emphasis placed on information giving, teaching and providing psychological support Orem's delineation of nursing actions may be used to describe interventions within the care pathway:

- Acting for or doing for another
- Guiding and directing
- Providing physical or psychological support
- Providing and maintaining an environment that supports personal development
- Teaching

The supportive-educative nursing action would have particular resonance in this situation. Peplau's (1952, 1991) suggestion that the nurse–patient relationship or partnership develops across admission, intervention, recovery and discharge also resonates within this particular environment. The supportive-educative nursing action would have particular resonance in this situation. Peplau's (1952, 1991) suggestion that the nurse-patient relationship or partnership develops across admission, intervention, recovery and discharge also resonates within this particular environment. By perhaps embracing this latter theory within care pathways, possibly integrating elements of another conceptual models, an alternative hybrid option may emerge that is sensitive to the needs of care pathway developers who are committed to retaining not only the nursing focus but the patient focus.

Conclusion

Contemporary day surgery holds particular challenges not only for nurses but for the whole multidisciplinary team. Internationally, in developed countries, there is an ever-increasing impetus to provide and perform increased numbers of short-stay surgeries, with the incumbent requirement for responsive day surgery facilities and staff. The nurse in this situation is known to multitask, both preparing and discharging patients who present for a range of surgeries. Ever concerned with quality care and increasingly aiming towards seamless multidisciplinary care, it is likely that internationally acclaimed care pathways will find favour within day surgery settings. Although minimally present within the international literature, the day surgery care pathway finds a particular home within the NHS (NHS 2008a) providing a rich resource for those thinking of embarking upon this route. While comprehensive in terms of total care delivery, care pathways could lead towards depersonalisation of patients and this should be avoided as this is not their intention. Rather their aim is to improve quality care. The patients' emotional experiences both prior to surgery and later within the hospital experience may take a lesser priority as a less tangible element of pathway delivery. However contemporary writers in the area are united in their claim that day surgery nurses must embrace the psychosocial element of patient care delivery. To this end, revisiting conceptual model based care may provide some of the philosophical elements necessary to guide *generalised* approaches to nursing care. By contextualising day surgery unit beliefs within one particular conceptual model or a conjoint model, nurses may begin to augment care pathway or other approaches. Furthermore, specific elements of the care pathway such as information giving, emotional reactions, pain and other adverse symptoms may be encapsulated within nursing language associated with conceptual model use and provide for a more comprehensive care plan in these areas, that can be still subjected to variance recording.

References

Alligood, M.R. and Marriner-Tomey, A. (2002a) Introduction to nursing theory: History, terminology, and analysis is practice. In: *Nursing Theorists and Their Work* (eds M.R. Alligood and A. Marriner-Tomey), 5th edn. Mosby, London.

Alligood, M.R. and Marriner-Tomey, A. (2002b) (eds) *Nursing Theorists and Their Work*, 5th edn. Mosby, London.

Berbiglia, V.A. (2002) Orem's self-care deficit nursing theory in practice. In: *Nursing Theorists and Their Work* (eds M.R. Alligood and A. Marriner-Tomey), 5th edn. Mosby, London.

Bergström, T., Carlson, T. and Jonson, A. (2000) Nursing care for ambulatory day surgery: The concept and organization of nursing care. *Ambulatory Surgery*, 8 (1), 3–5.

Campbell, H., Hotchkiss, R., Bradshaw, N. and Porteous, M. (1998) Integrated care pathways. *British Medical Journal*, 316, 133–7.

Coll, A.M. and Ameen, J. (2006) Profiles of pain after day surgery: Patients' experience of three different operation types. *Journal of Advanced Nursing*, 53 (2), 178–87.

Cormack, D.F.S. and Reynolds, W. (1992) Criteria for evaluating the clinical and practical utility of models used by nurses. *Journal of Advanced Nursing*, 17, 1472–8.

Costa, M.J. (2001) The lived perioperative experience of ambulatory surgery patients. *AORN Journal*, 74 (6), 874–81.

De Luc, K. (2000) Care pathways: An evaluation of their effectiveness. *Journal of Advanced Nursing*, 32 (2), 485–96.

Department of Health (1998a) *The New NHS: Modern, Dependable*. The Stationery Office, London.

Department of Health (1998b) *Commissioning in the New NHS*. Health Service Circular 198. Department of Health, Leeds.

Evers, G. (2002) Developing nursing science in Europe. *Journal of Nursing Scholarship*, 35 (1), 9–13.

Fawcett, J. (1995) *Analysis and evaluation of Conceptual Models of Nursing*, 3rd edn. F.A. Davies Company, Philadelphia.

Fawcett, J. (1999) The state of nursing science: Hallmarks of the 20th and 21st centuries. *Nursing Science Quarterly*, 12 (4), 311–4.

Fisher, A. and McMillan, R. (2004) *Integrated Care Pathways for Day Surgery*. Colman Print, Norwich.

Gilmartin, J. and Wright, K. (2007) The nurse's role in day surgery: A literature review. *International Nursing Review*, 54 (2), 183–90.

Graeme, A. (2000) A post-modern nursing model. *Nursing Standard*, 14 (34), 40–2.

Griffiths, P. (1998) An investigation into the description of patients' problems by nurses using two different needs-based nursing models. *Journal of Advanced Nursing*, 28 (5), 969–77.

Hodge, D. (1999) *Day Surgery: A Nursing Approach*. Churchill Livingstone, Edinburgh.

Holt, P., Wilson, A. and Ward, J. (1996) *Clinical Practice Guidelines and Critical Pathways: A Status Report on National and NSW Development and Implementation Activity*. NSW Health Department, Sydney.

Howard-Harwood, B. (1997) Care of the patient in the day surgical unit. In: *Day Surgery for Nurses* (ed L. Markanday). Whurr, London.

Hyde, A., Treacy M., Scott, A., MacNeela P., Butler M., Drennan J., Irving K., Byrne A. and Byrne, A. (2006) Social regulation, medicalisation and the nurse's role: Insights form a an analysis of nursing documentation. *International Journal of Nursing Studies*, 43 (6), 735–44.

Inatavicius, D.D. and Hausmann, K.A. (1995) *Clinical Pathways for Collaborative Practice.* W.B. Saunders Company, Philadelphia.

James, D. (2000) Patients' perceptions of day surgery. *British Journal of Perioperative Nursing*, 10 (9), 466–72.

Johnson, S. (1997a) What is a pathway of care? In: *Pathways of Care*, (ed S. Johnson). Blackwell Science, Oxford.

Johnson, S. (1997b) (ed) *Pathways of Care.* Blackwell Science, Oxford.

Kitchiner D., Davidson C. and Bundred P. (1996) Integrated care pathways: Effective tools of continuous evaluation of clinical practice. *Journal of Evaluation in Clinical Practice*, 2, 65–9.

Kitson, K. (2007) Bunions: Their origin and treatment. *Journal of Perioperative Practice*, 17 (7), 308–10, 315–6.

McCabe, C. and Timmins, F. (2006) *Communication Skills for Nursing Practice.* Palgrave Macmillan, London.

McClune, B. and Franklin, K. (1987) The Mead model for nursing: Adapted from the Roper/Logan/Tierney model for nursing. *Intensive Care Nursing*, 3, 97–103.

Mitchell, M. (1997) Patients' perceptions of pre-operative preparation for day surgery. *Journal of Advanced Nursing*, 26 (2), 356–63.

Mitchell, M. (2000) Anxiety management: A distinct nursing role in day surgery. *Journal of Ambulatory Surgery*, 8 (3), 119–27.

Mitchell, M. (2003) Patient and modern and elective surgery: A literature review. *Journal of Clinical Nursing*, 12, 806–15.

Mitchell, M. (2006) Nursing knowledge and the expansion of day surgery in the United Kingdom. *Journal of Ambulatory Surgery*, 12, 131–8.

Mitchell, M. (2007) Constructing information booklets for day-case patients. *Ambulatory Surgery*, 9, 37–45.

Marriner-Tomey, A. (2000) Foreword. In: Roper, N., Logan, W.W. and Tierney, A.J. (2001) *The Roper Logan Tierney Model of Nursing Based on Activities of Living.* Churchill Livingstone, London.

Mason, C. (1999) Guide to practice or 'load of rubbish'? The influence of care plans on nursing practice in five clinical areas in Northern Ireland. *Journal of Advanced Nursing*, 29 (2), 380–87.

Murphy, K., Cooney, A., Casey, D., Connor, M., O'Connor, J. and Dineen, B. (2000) The Roper, Logan and Tierney Model: Perceptions and operationalization of the model in psychiatric nursing within one health board in Ireland. *Journal of Advanced Nursing*, 31 (6), 1333–41.

National Council for the Professional Development of Nursing and Midwifery (NCNM) (2006) *Improving the Patient Journey: Understanding Integrated Care Pathways.* NCNM, Dublin.

National Health Service (NHS) (2005) Quality Improvement Scotland (2005) Clinical Governance & Risk Management: Achieving safe, effective, patient-focused care and services NHS Quality Improvement, Scotland.

National Health Service (NHS) (2008a) Protocols & Care Pathways Specialist Library Online. http:// www.library.nhs.uk/pathways (accessed 1 February 2008).

National Health Service (NHS) (2008b) *National Library for Health* Online. http:// www.library.nhs.uk (accessed 29 August 2008).

Orem, D.E. (1971, 1980, 1985, 1995, 2001) *Nursing: Concepts of Practice*, 1st, 2nd, 3rd, 4th, 5th & 6th edn. Mosby, London.

Otte, D. (1996) Patients' perspectives and experiences of day surgery. *Journal of Advanced Nursing*, 23 (6), 1228–37.

Peplau, H.E. (1952, 1991) *Interpersonal Relations in Nursing*. MacMillan Education, London.

Pearson, A, Vaughan B. and Fitzgerald M. (2001) *Nursing Models for Practice*, 2nd edn. Butterworth Heinemann, London.

Renholm, M., Leino-Kilpi, H., Suominen, T. (2002) Critical pathways: A systematic review. *Journal of Nursing Administration*, 32 (4), 196–202.

Riley, K. (1998) Paving the way. *Health Service Journal*, 108, 30–1.

Rogan Foy, C. and Timmins, F. (2004) Improving communication in day surgery settings. *Nursing Standard*, 17 (9), 37–43.

Roper, N., Logan, W.W. and Tierney, A.J. (1980, 1985, 1990, 1996) *The Elements of Nursing A Model for Nursing Based on a Model for Living*, 1st, 2nd, 3rd & 4th edn. Churchill Livingstone, London.

Shamsudin, N. (2002) Can the Newman systems model be adapted to the Malaysian nursing context? *International Journal of Nursing Practice*, 8, 99–105.

Stead, L. and Huckle, S. (1997) Pathways in cardiology. In: *Pathways of Care*, (ed S. Johnson). Blackwell Science, Oxford.

Susilahti, H., Suominen, T. and Leino-Kilpi, H. (2004) Recovery of Finnish short-stay surgery patients *Medsurg Nursing*, 13 (5), 326–35.

Sutcliffe, L. (1994) Philosophy and models in critical care nursing. *Intensive and Critical Care Nursing*, 10, 212–21.

Taylor, S.G., Geden, E., Issaramalai, S. and Wongvatunyu, S. (2000) Orem's Self-Care Deficit Nursing Theory: Its philosophic foundation and the state of the science. *Nursing Science Quarterly* 13 (2), 104–108.

Thompson, D. (2002) Nurse-directed services: How can they be made more effective? *European Journal of Cardiovascular Nursing*, 1, 7–10.

Tierney, A.J (1998) Nursing Models extant or extinct? *Journal of Advanced Nursing*, 8 (1), 77–85.

Timmins, F. (2005) *Contemporary Issues in Coronary Care Nursing*. Routledge, London.

Townsend, R. and Cox, F. (2007) Standardised analgesia packs after day case orthopaedic surgery. *The Journal of Perioperative Practice*, 17 (7), 340–6.

Treacy, P. and Hyde, A. (2003) Developments in Nursing in Republic of Ireland: The emergence of a disciplinary discourse. *Journal of Professional Nursing*, 19 (2), 91–8.

Wall, D. and Proyect, M.M. (1998) *Moving from Parameters to Pathways: A Guide for Developing and Implementing Critical Pathways*. Precept Press, Chicago.

Nurse-led Pre-admission Clinics

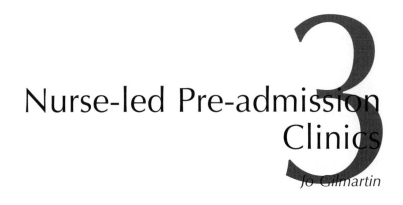

Jo Gilmartin

Introduction

Globally day surgery has increased significantly in developed countries, representing 50–80% of all surgical procedures (Pearson et al. 2004). Expanding day surgery is number one in the '10 High Impact Changes' suggested as part of the NHS Modernisation Agenda (NHS Modernisation Agency 2004). The NHS plan (DH 2000) anticipates facilitating three-quarters of all surgical operations as a day surgery procedure by 2010. Pre-operative assessment is a vital component to ensure that patients are appropriately selected, informed and prepared (Smith et al. 2006). Nurse-run pre-assessment clinics (PAC) facilitate these processes. The nurse's role in contemporary day surgery is evolving in the form of multiskilling enabling the workforce to rotate within various areas of day surgery (Cooke et al. 2004). This chapter, then, is concerned with the emergence of nurse-led interventions; the centrality of nurse-led pre-admission clinics, the challenge of setting up a nurse-led clinic and evaluating services.

The emergence of nurse-led interventions

Pre-assessment is an evolving concept, gaining momentum in the USA in the 1970s and becoming acknowledged and valued in the UK in the 1980s. The move to day surgery in the UK was inspired by the *Guidelines for Day Case*

Surgery (1985) produced by the Royal College of Surgeons and this was modified in 1992. This report enthused the development of day surgery indicating that it was 'the best option for 50% for patients undergoing elective procedures' (Jackson 2007: 177). Moreover the significance of pre-assessment was also emphasised, in an attempt to reduce cancellations and align with government targets. In the UK the British Association of Day Surgery (BADS) was created in 1989 to encourage the development of day surgery promoting the provision of quality.

The drive to day surgery was strongly emphasised in the NHS plan (DH 2000) in an attempt to reduce elective surgical waiting times and promote patient-centred care. Pre-operative assessment has been advocated as an intervention to achieve this intent (Bramhall 2002). A further major initiative to enhance the government's commitment to pre-operative assessment was the Operating Theatre and Pre-operative Assessment Programme that was formed (NHS Modernisation Agency 2004) with the goal of reducing the number of cancelled operations and waiting times. An enthusiastic attempt to standardise pre-operative testing was produced by NICE (2003) with the emergence of guidelines for practitioners.

Doctor-nurse substitute

Effective pre-assessment is a crucial element to ensure that selection criteria are applied rigorously. Historically junior doctors have undertaken this role. The growth of postgraduate medical training (NHS management Executive 1993) combined with the initiative in the UK to reduce junior doctors workloads (NHS management Executive 1991) impacted significantly on the time that doctors were available to meet NHS requirement. These changes were also driven by efficiency savings, and with dynamic initiatives to substitute nurses for preregistration house officers (Richardson et al. 1995). This shift brought new challenges to nurses to embrace new, exciting roles. Nevertheless, the engagement with new, extended roles seemed to render nurses inferior in the traditionally doctor-dominated domain. The culturally assumed difference between the relative abilities of doctors and nurses was problematic for some nurses. For instance, a feeling of transgression appeared to be associated with the very act of thinking a new role – created by doctors. More specifically, medical perceptions of assessment (Smith 2007) are often at variance with nurses' perceptions. Such a figuration could powerfully represent or signify contrasting orientations. Crucially, clear guidelines and selection criteria protocols are vital. The presence of such descriptions could assume a linguistic function, which might impact on interpretation and utilisation. These multiple issues posit huge challenges, potentially impacting on the pre-assessment process.

In recognition of role change, the expanding role of nurse practitioners since the 1980s extended its remit to integrating physical examination skills into assessment strategies (Walgrove 2004). The incorporation of this intervention, in conjunction with history taking, problem solving and the ability to collaborate with other health professionals equipped nurses to undertake holistic assessments. The growth of new nursing roles was encouraged too by the government's strategic planning. Nurses in day surgery developed a distinct, multiskilled role, which is sometimes referred to as the extended specialist-nursing role (Mitchell 2000b). The new role enabled nurses to make a real difference to the psychological care of patients, by engaging with anxiety management in the pre- and post-operative stages (Mitchell, 2000b). In a randomised controlled trial (RCT) undertaken by Kinley et al. (2002), it was highlighted that appropriately trained nurses are not inferior to preregistration house officers in carrying out pre-operative assessments. The sample involved 1874 patients; 926 were assessed by house officers and 948 by nurses. The results showed that house officers ordered more unnecessary investigations than the trained nurses, who adhered to the protocol more than house officers.

The epistemological debate about the ontology of nursing and whether the scope of professional practice develop internally is questioned by Coyler (2004). Operational frameworks for nurse practitioners emphasise functional roles such as dynamic practice, professional efficacy, clinical leadership and a legislative structure for extended practice (Gardener et al. 2006). Personal attributes and significant communication skills are not emphasised. This is further compounded by a scarcity of high-level evidence (Muir Gray 2001) related to desired skill-mix and staffing models in day surgery units (Pearson et al. 2004). The recommended optimal staffing levels in day surgery are drawn from expert opinion rather than systematic inquiry (Gilmartin and Wright 2007).

Impetus for role change

A further major impetus for role change and development appeared to be linked with shifts in social relationships, the postmodern culture birthing and promoting individualism and empowerment. This shift paved the way for holistic theories about health and wellbeing, moving away from the biomedical model of care, with the intent to improve intervention for individual patients. This resulted in greater awareness of patient expectation about information, choice of treatment options and waiting times. Most of these changes enabled non-medical professionals to spearhead key roles in facilitating care and treatment interventions within the context of patient-centred services. Government response to social change, outlining declarations for making a difference (DH 1999a, 1999b), (NHS Modernisation Agency 2004) led to the development of key roles for nurses and higher levels of nursing practice. This has created the opportunity for a substantial increase in clinical nurse specialists (CNSs), nurse practitioners (NPs), advanced nurse practitioners (APNs) and consultant nurses (CNs), particularly in the UK (Lloyd-Jones 2005) and at an international level.

Multiskilled roles

Currently in the UK nurses working in a day surgery context undertake multiskilled roles. Drawing on Mitchell's view (2005), this involves initiating several aspects of care from pre-assessment to admission, moving on to perioperative phase, to recovery and discharge planning. The pre-assessment in particular requires a comprehensive approach, ensuring that social, medical and psychological variables are assessed and co-morbidies are known (Smith 2007). Mitchell (2005: 182) goes on to suggest that the evolving a multiskilled role might be linked to competency rating, for example, capacity to 'perform tasks such as venepuncture, cannulation and read electrocardiographs (ECGs)'. The innovation aligned with the extended role is not only attributed to the devolution of medical tasks. Professional knowledge and nursing skills also contribute to effective nursing intervention (RCN 2002), especially in the pre-assessment stage (Gilmartin 2004). However, the label 'multiskilled role' has been service driven to fill in gaps created by shortages and changes to medical staff roles and public expectation.

Functional role descriptions are lacking in explicit ontological foundations and 'can be transposed into tasks and divorced from the value bases which guide particular professions' approaches to care giving' (Coyler 2004, p.410),

This results in the evolvement of competency frameworks that provide measurable standards for practitioner performance, perhaps assessed and fitted into a job evaluation category. Competency frameworks are indeed useful and attractive but potentially they might downplay the expertise needed to facilitate complex care. One major role of nurse practitioners in the pre-assessment clinic is assessing patient suitability, which can be potentially challenging. The pre-assessment intervention is strongly influenced by medical protocols transposed into operational tasks for nurses.

The disarrays of ontology

The redefinition is advantageous in functional terms, assuring medical fitness for day surgery (Smith 2007), however, the ontology of nursing has lost ground in the construction of multiskilling and extended roles. The utilisation of a reductionist approach has been shaped by government initiatives and medical influence. Nevertheless, nursing knowledge and evidence-based practice is gaining momentum in influencing nurse-led pre-assessment, anxiety management, information giving and pre-and post-operative care. The growth of nursing knowledge for modern surgery is also encouraged by Mitchell (2006), suggesting that nurse educators need to develop flexible educational programmes linked to evolving roles. To enable proper professional expertise to prevail, nurse-led intervention requires a strong ontological base in conjunction with functional characteristics. Thus, to follow the desire of disciplinary belongings and aspirations is fundamental to the evolving role.

What is clear from the RCN (2002) guidelines is that nurse practitioners require preparation at degree level. Moreover, a higher level of academic preparation (Read et al. 2000), such as study at Master's level, is important for advanced practice roles. Crucially, without accreditation, adequate educational preparation and assessment of competence, nurses and their employers are vulnerable to litigation (Marsden et al. 2007). There is a danger that new roles could be reactive and random, being compromised by jumbled planning and economic constraints. Nurses involved in pre-assessment have a vital role to play in understanding the centrality of education for role expansion and be prepared to argue and advocate for it.

Nurse-led services

The majority of nurses spearheading nurse-led services are innovative, advanced practitioners, facilitating the quiet revolution of more effective, patient-centred care. Nurse-led pre-admissions clinics were developed in the 1980s and have been enthused further by the Modernisation Agenda (NHS Modernisation Agency 2004). They were introduced to improve pre-operative assessment, reduce elective surgical waiting times and cancelled operations, and promote patient-centred care. The government encouraged these initiatives through the Modernisation Agency's Operating Theatre and Pre-operative Assessment Programme, which was completed in 2004. The major aspiration of this particular project was to reduce waiting times for surgery and cancelled operations. Practice development was inspired, too, by NICE guidelines (2003) for pre-operative testing, with the intent of standardising services across the UK.

Patient selection usually begins at outpatient clinics with medical staff, referring potential patients to the day surgical unit for pre-admission assessment. The pre-assessment process is led by suitably trained nurse practitioners. Not surprisingly, the development and ethos of pre-assessment clinics vary, from those entirely nurse-led (Gilmartin 2004), to those with significant leadership from the anaesthetic department, to others with a medical input (Connolly 2003, Smith et al. 2006). Crucially, nurse-led clinics require competent nurses with the capacity to undertake comprehensive assessments and work at the interface with allied professionals.

The 'one stop shop'

Some nurse-led pre-admission clinics are accredited practice development units, others are multidisciplinary services; there tends to be a lack of uniformity in service provision in the UK (Walgrove 2004). Arguably, practice development should incorporate a range of approaches and is greatly influenced by the creativity of practitioners and the integration of local contextual issues (Page 2002). Practise development usually evolves over time and the process is greatly influenced by team innovation, evidence-based practice and quality improvement (Chin and Hamer 2006). Cost-efficiency drives and streamlining have encouraged nurse-led services to spearhead a 'one stop pre-assessment and treatment' where patients are immediately pre-assessed for day surgery after an outpatient consultation.

This is often considered the gold standard (Karthikeyan et al. 2007), being hugely beneficial to patients in terms of time management, because an additional attendance to hospital prior to surgery is not required; beneficial outcomes, such as greater patient satisfaction, resource utilisation and cost reduction, further highlight the legitimacy of pre-assessment units. In spite of efficiency drives, Karthikeyan et al. (2007: 257) reported that some patients who attended the 'one stop shop' would have preferred more time to consider undergoing an operation before signing the consent form. They recommend a 'deferment to think about the surgery' for patients wishing for more time, with a two week period for reflection and decision-making.

Integration of services

Assessing patient's fitness for surgery often involves a varied range of tests. Most nurse-led units also have the capacity to offer a range of services. In the process of screening, patients can undergo ECGs, chest x-rays, and blood tests and access a pharmacist if required. There are also facilities for Meticillin-resistant Staphylococcus aureus (MRSA) screening which is important in pre-operative surgical patients (DH 2006a). Accessing a range of services in one unit is beneficial to patients, reducing time spent travelling to other departments for specific tests.

Additionally, nurses provide information and education, utilise creative ways to explore the reduction of pre-operative anxiety, and address lifestyle management and health promotion. Empirical evidence confirms patient benefits and satisfaction regarding the pre-assessment intervention. Patients have reported a reduction in anxiety; increased confidence and a greater understanding of perioperative care arrangements (Clark et al. 2000: 95). Other studies also emphasise a reduction in anxiety, success in knowledge gained about the day surgery experience and parent and child satisfaction (O'Shea 2007).

What are the significant features of selection criteria?

To promote better outcomes for patients, it is essential that pre-assessment nurses work with protocols and guidelines, which have been developed locally. The selection criteria are usually defined and collaboratively agreed by the anaesthetists, surgeons and nurses involved in day surgery. Criteria protocols and guidelines are strongly influenced by the NICE (2003) pre-operative tests, outlining grades associated with fitness to undergo anaesthesia. In addition, the *Good Practice Guide to Day Surgery* (2005) http://www.doh.gov.uk (day surgery section), *Day Surgery Operational Guide* (RCN 2002), BADS (2006) *Directory of Procedure*, suggesting achievable target rates with a list of 160 operations, are helpful. Pre-admission assessment guidelines (Box 3.1) to maximise efficiency are also put forward by Cooke et al. (2005).

Due to the expansion of day surgery targets the selection criteria require broadening (Smith 2007) to match the planned procedures. This is crucial to prevent cancellations, to ensure that co-morbidities are recognised, treated and patients are well informed and prepared for day surgery. Arguably, discrepancy in protocols could lead to deficits in pre-operative assessment and cancellations. A ten-year observational study of cancellations in day surgery undertaken by Jiménez et al. (2006) highlighted reasons such as acute medical conditions, patient decisions to refuse and failure to follow pre-operative guidelines. Therefore in attempting to achieve day surgery targets (Cooke et al. 2004) it is vital to follow current protocols.

A fairly recent systematic review of the 'Best Practice' in day surgery (Pearson et al. 2004) described two effective interventions in relation to the pre-admission care of patients. The first related to pre-operative telephone

---

Box 3.1   Domains of pre-assessment

Domains of pre-assessment

- Follow a pre-agreed protocol
- Include suitability of the condition for day surgery
- Assess patient fitness
- Assess home circumstances for discharge
- Inform the patient about the procedure
- Allow time for the patient to reflect and ask questions
- Consider age since adverse factors may increase with age
- Familiarise patients with day surgery environment
- Educate the patient and carers about surgery and post-operative care

screening or questionnaire and the second to a pre-admission appointment a few days prior to admission. Now, however, face-to-face screening a few weeks prior to surgery is preferable, allowing appropriate tests to be carried out and reviewed and thus ensuring that patients are adequately prepared and treatments are optimised on the day of surgery itself. It is essential that protocols be developed for patients who request to postpone and re-book procedures for compelling reasons (Smith et al. 2006). These protocols would enables the re-allocation of procedure slots instantaneously in the day unit, encouraging efficient use of resources.

The pre-assessment process

The pre-assessment interview is a vital part of day surgery. The nurse involved is required to undertake a rigorous assessment, being alert to underlying problems, because some patients might not disclose the whole story. Independent risk factors for both surgery and anaesthesia such as obesity and or cardiac problems need to be evaluated carefully. Assessment documentation is usually designed by local Trusts and, to facilitate a holistic assessment, nurses could utilise a framework such as Orem's Self-Care Deficit Nursing Theory (SCDNT) (Orem, 1971, 1980, 1985, 1995, 2001).

The concept of self-care is mainly connected with a desire to allow patients to take the initiative and be responsible for their own health where possible. This has consequences for the nurse's role, in terms of enhancing the self-care abilities of the patient (Chang 1980). When conducting a pre-assessment interview, apart from problem identification, the primary focus is assessing the care demands of the patient and their capacity to meet self-care demands independently. This might include activities such as physical exercise, positive nutritional practices, or goals directed at promoting high levels of wellbeing, in the preparation for surgery. Arguably, patient involvement in decision-making and goal-setting is a crucial step in achieving successful self-care.

The nature of nurse–patient interactions

Dynamic communication is a key factor in facilitating a successful pre-assessment interview. Communication in day surgery settings will be further discussed in Chapter 7, however it is important to note at this point that the quality of the nurse–patient interaction within nurse-led pre-admission services relies on the capacity of nurse practitioners to build rapport, gather information, inform patients about procedure, educate, challenge and empower. To facilitate therapeutic communication, being genuine, open, non-judgemental and displaying empathy is imperative (Rogers 1980). The significance of sustained, positive interactions with patients is fundamental (Rogan and Timmins 2004). Rogan and Timmins (2004) suggest that – while noting the verbal utterances, para-language and non-verbal cues displayed by the patient – active listening is a vital ingredient.

Paralinguistics might be a central feature in pre-assessment: 'hesitations', 'prolonged pauses' or voice tone might suggest that the patient is emotionally distressed, 'shutting down', or resisting key questions and not disclosing the whole story. To sustain and open up dialogue, supportive responding skills and sensitive questioning is paramount. Attunement is also a significant characteristic; this requires the nurse to harness synchrony and symmetry in communication, displaying a capacity to match the mood and intensity of emotion disclosed by the patient, which gives a sense of psychological connection (Stern 1985; Cortina and Marrone, 2003). For instance, a patient might disclose intense anxiety about the anticipated day surgery procedure. This type of disclosure requires a dynamic, emphatic response, permitting the patient to get in touch and talk about their state in more depth. Each patient is idiosyncratic and so nurse practitioners need to be equipped with a sophisticated range of communication skills (McCabe and Timmins 2006) (Box 3.2) to undertake a comprehensive pre-assessment interview.

Box 3.2   Communication skills

Communication skills

Giving clear information
Active listening
Empathic responses
Using open and closed questions
Observing non-verbal communication
Attunement
Prompting

Reflecting

Clarifying
Checking understanding
Paraphrasing

Challenging
Summarising

Ending

(Egan 2002; McCabe and Timmins 2006)

Although nurse practitioners' professional knowledge and communication competencies have been expanded (RCN 2002) to include the development of counselling skills, there is some research evidence to suggest that deficits in nurse-patient communication prevail. Williams et al. (2003) showed that patients felt dissatisfied with information provision; they were not offered any explanation about the surgical procedure and did not know who their surgeon was. In contrast Scott (2001) highlighted that 89.5% who received information said they found it 'just right'; nonetheless, 22% of the patients telephoned the hospital for further information prior to admission. Rhodes et al. (2006:184) revealed that participants were 'inadequately informed about the procedure, fearful of losing control both physically and psychologically, and nurses either dismissed or inadequately dealt with their fears of anaesthesia and surgery.'

In the context of pre-assessment, different modes of information delivery can be utilised. This could include: video clips or DVDs displaying diverse day surgery procedures and different types of anaesthesia interventions; creative, written information on procedures; or verbal instruction from nurses. Crucially, verbal information needs to be simplified and made specific about details, using reinforcement techniques (Rogan and Timmins 2004). To prevent communication breakdown, checking understanding is essential and this type of intervention enables the patient to reflect to ask questions and seek further clarification if required.

In a multicultural society some patients may not be fluent in English and may feel unable to participate fully in the pre-assessment interview. The major factor here is to determine whether or not assessment can be performed without interpreter intervention. At the outset, it would be very worthwhile to undertake an assessment of language need (Boyle and Andrews 2003) to identify the appropriate interpreter match. Gender issues and confidentiality are also important variables to consider when arranging interpreting services. Patients will feel far better supported, far less alone, if sustained attempts are made to meet language need, enabling them to participate more fully in pre-assessment interview and thus leading to greater patient satisfaction.

Acute assessment intervention

Pre-assessment is a thorough process, facilitating the immediate identification of the social, physical and psychological aspects of patients' needs. Building rapport is essential from the outset. Recognition can be accomplished in a simple act of greeting or by the employment of attending and responding skills. Although verbal introjects are particularly valuable, the profoundest step of recognition is through non-verbal cues, such as sensitive eye contact. Collaboration, an important characteristic that allows the patient to use their initiative and abilities, can be achieved by explaining the purpose of the interview, encouraging the patient to actively engage, and permitting the nurse and patient to work together in an expansive way. Casting the patient in an active role puts power in their hands.

Facilitation is a helpful intervention and enables the interview to get started. Here a subtle and gentle imagination comes into play. There is a readiness to respond to the gesture, which a patient makes, enabling inter-personal action to occur.

When this is done well, there is great sensitivity to the patient's verbal utterances and interaction proceeds at a speed that is convivial to the patient. In some instances, carers might be present merging with the inter-view interaction as meaning develops. Acknowledging and validating a carer's contribution is vital: this helps to connect them with the reality of the pre-assessment process. The task of facilitation involves a high degree of empathy if a patient's holistic frame of reference is to be understood.

The dynamic process

Assessment is a step-by-step and meticulous. The process of making a valid approximation of patient fitness, benefits and risks of day surgery is driven by a pre-agreed protocol, aligned with Orem's model, which provides a considerable capacity to identify social, psychological and physical health care deficits which can be met prior to admission for day surgery. Through-out the assessment process, the use of open questions is significant, to allow full elaboration about immediate need and chronic conditions if prevalent, such as diabetes, asthma, hypertension or epilepsy. For example, diabetic patients need to be screened 'to identify co-existing cardiovascular, renal or autonomic dysfunction' (Smith 2007: 185). This usually requires blood tests and electrocardiogram (ECG). A physical examination may also be under-taken and if, for example, a heart murmur is present, further investigations such as an echocardiogram might be required. Patient intervention should be preceded by informed consent. Discussion with the patient should reflect a rationale for the test, the implications of normal and abnormal results, including benefits or risks to the surgical procedure. It is also useful to establish if the patient is taking any prescribed medication, herbal or homeo-pathic remedies, or has any specific allergies.

Health risks

Hypertension and obesity also present challenges. Smith (2007) argues that if hypertension is suspected at pre-assessment, and surgical intervention is not urgent, patients can be referred for further assessment. In the UK, a body mass index (BMI) of 30 or above is classified as obese, over 35 is known as morbid obesity, and over 40 indicate extreme obesity (DH 2007).

However, BMI is calculated according to the western body. In the context of a more general process of globalisation, obesity is epidemic and is clearly affecting countries such as China and The Gambia. The specific application of a standard BMI might be flawed because of typical differences such as bone density. Current British guidelines point to a body mass index of <35 kg as acceptable for day surgery, if no other contraindications are present. Nevertheless, a body mass index of 35–40 kg should be acceptable (NHS Modernisation Agency 2002). Canadian anaesthetists appear to be more liberal, with a willingness to accept patients with BMI of 35–44 kg and sometimes above, provided they are in good health (Friedman et al. 2003). Smith (2007) goes on to suggest that it is essential not to consider BMI in isolation from other significant variables, such as type of surgical intervention, general fitness and smoking, which might increase risks related to obesity.

Social issues

Social assessment is important because patients presenting for day surgery should have a responsible adult who is fit and willing to care for them for the first 24 hours. It is appropriate to begin discharge planning at the pre-assessment, identifying challenges (Gilmartin 2007), constraints or support mechanisms. A considerable number of people live alone in developed countries; less developed countries appear to have robust family networks, which are a huge advantage in a day surgery context, particularly in relation to aftercare provision (Gilmartin and Wright 2007). Elderly patients may not have suitable carers, and patients with small children will require extra help for a few days. With sufficient planning, the majority will be able to organise a relative or friend to help or stay with a family member for a few days. Long journeys or air travel are best avoided immediately after surgery (Smith 2007); facilities for emergency care should be accessible at the home destination.

Psychological wellbeing

Emphasis should be placed on careful psychological assessment to elicit actual or potential fears or anxieties. For example, a patient might share concerns about undertaking the procedure, asserting:

- 'I feel frightened and anxious about having a general anaesthetic.'
- 'Worrying thoughts go through my mind about the operation.'
- 'I get 'butterflies' in my stomach when I think about the procedure.'

Validation and attunement are useful responding skills to employ, acknowledging the reality and power of the patient's emotions and feelings.

Validation permits the person to feel connected, alive and in touch with feeling state, even if it is chaotic or suspicious. This type of intervention needs to be interspersed with giving information about the procedure or the anaesthetic, encouraging the patient to ask questions and explore concerns in greater depth. Careful documentation of the information gathered during the pre-assessment interview is essential (NHS Modernisation Agency 2002), to facilitate problem identification and the construction of a care plan. The plan might involve educational intervention, lifestyle management, or techniques for anxiety reduction, which will be explored in the following section.

Educational intervention

This is a top priority, because patients undergoing day surgery need to be provided with clear information about the procedure, the day of surgery itself and the aftercare. Another important contribution might relate to health education, or education in regard to medication, pain management, or ways of reducing anxiety (Box 3.3). Alongside information provision, it came to be recognised that there are many ways in which evidence-based practice could be incorporated into pre-operative education. For example, the use of music in reducing pre-operative anxiety (Lee et al. 2004; Cooke et al. 2005). Here there is a dramatic shift towards empowering patients to self-care. As the concern to provide effective pre-operative education has grown, it has been increasingly recognised that there is a need for quality standards and for sound methods of teaching. Arguably, there is a dearth of evidence to determine the efficacy of pre-operative educational intervention in day surgery.

Box 3.3   Educational Activity

Educational Activity

What does the day surgery procedure entail?
What are the benefits of day surgery?
What happens on the day of surgery itself?
Who can I contact if I require further information before admission?
What techniques might be helpful to reduce anxiety?
How can I improve my wellbeing prior to surgery?
What websites provide the 'best' information about day surgery?
How might I cope with nausea or pain following the procedure?
How might I prepare for discharge?
What does the carer's role involve?

In spite of research deficits, it is crucial that pre-assessment nurses consider factors that influence pre-operative education and how it is managed in everyday practice. The focus will vary, depending on individual needs of patients and carers. Creativity is a vital ingredient in the use of diverse methods to facilitate the 'best' approach, including group lectures if appropriate, one-to-one teaching, the use of booklets or pamphlets, video clips, audiovisual presentations or DVDs, or a amalgamation of one or more teaching method. For example, 'a booklet containing bright pictures and simple, child-friendly explanatory text' (O'Shea 2007: 49) combined with video viewing appear to be powerful tools in the preparation of children for day surgery.

The majority of pre-assessment clinics provide written materials to support verbal instruction. In relation to day surgery procedures, written information often carries meaning of a biomedical nature (Mitchell 2006). Further deficits in information leaflets for flexible cystoscopy was emphasised by Shah et al. (2007), suggesting that leaflets need to contain more vital, accurate and up-to-date information. Of course information will be impregnated with day surgery culture, meaning and values but accuracy, clarity and contemporary information is essential.

Educational activities may be facilitated by the pre-assessment nurse or by allied health professionals. A patient might be referred to a diabetic specialist, dietician, pharmacist or to the hypertension clinic. Educational outcomes are usually tailored to match individual circumstances. The significance of specialist input cannot be overestimated. For example, a pharmacist might be essential to consider chronic medication and the benefits of temporary suspension or the danger of stopping medication prior to surgery. Homeopathy and herbal medicine is becoming more popular; although most are benign (Smith 2007), some might have to be stopped prior to surgery.

Effects of music on anxiety

Educating patients about anxiety reduction is enthusiastically encouraged by evidence-based practice. Striking results revealed the usefulness of distraction to reduce pre-operative anxiety, displaying the highest level of evidence (level 1 Muir Gray 2001). Distraction was in the form of music and short stories delivered in personal stereo systems (Markland and Hardy 1993). This variable was also been emphasised by Lee et al. (2004) and Cooke et al. (2005). The physiological parameters for both the control and intervention groups were reduced significantly during the pre-procedure period (Lee et al. 2004). Moreover, only the intervention group who were provided with self–selected music had a remarkable reduction in reported anxiety levels. Recommendations were therefore made to administer self-selected music to day surgery patients.

Further evidence to support this view is also reported by Cooke et al. (2005). Pre- and post-test measures of anxiety were undertaken using the State-Trait Anxiety Inventory. The results revealed that music significantly reduced the state anxiety level of the intervention group. This is an important finding and provides clear evidence for the use of appropriate music in a day surgery context (Gilmartin and Wright 2007). The use of music may not be preferable for every patient, however. Specific intervention, personalised to individual need, is required for patients with anxiety problems.

Alternatively, patients can be encouraged to use EFT (Emotional Freedom Techniques) and energy psychology tools (Feinstein et al. 2005) This contemporary approach can help overcome a range of psychological problems such as fear, anxiety, guilt or shame promoting harmony and coherence.

Lifestyle Management

There are several different theories that offer legitimate and optimistic interventions for changing health beliefs and health behaviour (Kerr et al. 2005; Conner and Norman 2005). Nonetheless, changing health beliefs is often threatening. People troubled by smoking addictions or stressful lifestyles, or who are plagued by obesity, might have deep feelings of helplessness in controlling significant areas of their lives. Despite the challenges and resistance portrayed by patients, health professionals need to facilitate change with clarity and positive intention. To help patients shift beliefs and accomplish goals, Orem's Self-Care Deficit Theory (SCDT) might be useful.

Health promoting behaviour is usually congruent with Orem's (1971, 1980, 1985, 1995, 2001) ideas of self-care activity, which were alluded to in Chapter 2. Self-care involves the practice of activities that individuals initiate and practice on their own behalf. Health-promoting behaviours concord with Orem's philosophy, because they are concerned with health-related activities and purposeful action. Health promotion self-care appears to resonate with the construct of therapeutic self-care demand, which consists of three self-care requisites, including:

- Universal self-care requisites (USCR)
- Development self-care requisites (DSCR)
- Health deviation self-care requisites (HDSCR)

Interestingly, health promotion self-care is perceived as being an integral part of a person's lifestyle, with actions directed towards meeting selected USCR and DSCR. During the actual process of pre-assessment, deficits might come to the surface when there is some problem that needs special attention, such as sudden sleep interruption due to the impact of stress, and a set of self-care health goals need to be constructed to reduce stress, promote sleep and increase levels of wellbeing. Health deviation self-care requisites are required when the patient has a specific condition and or under medical care. For example, a patient with hypertension, diabetes or obesity might present with a specific deficit, meaning that health promotion activities and lifestyle management might need to be designed and negotiated by a specialist such as a dietician. Creativity and innovation is essential in enabling patients to sustain commitment to lifestyle changes.

The internet as a source of health information

The rapid growth in web-based health-care information has generated numerous sites focusing on 'health lifestyle' issues, some of which might be useful source for nurses involved in lifestyle management, particularly in regard to tacking obesity and encouraging physical activity. Some web sites include interactive features, physical activity advice, personalised progress charts, e-mail access to expert advice and local community activity. Although the internet is another facet of the paradigm shift in health care, the onerous challenge for health professionals is the credibility and trustworthiness of the information given at different web sites.

The notion of quality assessment and quality grading is crucial to empowering online health users to elicit reliable information. Many health sites have significant shortcomings, as the utilisation of scientifically-based criteria to assess them would be difficult (Korp 2005). Korp goes on to suggest that the quality of health information is associated with the trust people place in it. Of course, scientific standards of quality and trust are two distinct issues. Essentially, health professionals should attempt to construct a benchmark for good quality health information, empowering clients to make a distinction between useful and poor health information. User involvement could be inspirational in the identification of 'gold standard' web sites. Day surgery patients appear to have the capacity to self-care and could access credible web sites for information and knowledge relevant to lifestyle management.

Setting up a nurse-led pre-admission clinic

The case for better pre-assessment has become overwhelmingly strong. If we compare the standards and expectations of pre-assessment care (Macdonald et al. 1999) held almost ten years ago with those that are held today, the changes would seem almost revolutionary. The following section will offer brief practical advice on setting up a nurse-led clinic. This is a major practice development initiative, which receives greater elaboration in Chapter 4. In this period of history, when cost-effectiveness has been made into a fetish, practice development has to be filled by a model that grasps the meaning of streamlining and innovation. These ideas need to be developed and driven by a team of committed individuals moving towards the accreditation of practice.

The strategic task of developing a new service requires well-motivated, energetic and enthusiastic team players that are committed to the vision of the new service. Crucially, practice development is a patient-focused activity, influenced by policy, which is perceived as a synthesis of three discrete elements: quality improvement, evidence-based practice and innovation (Page and Hammer 2002). Clearly, careful thought needs to given to the way we integrate the three vital ingredients and how we expect different team members to work together. In addition, there maybe changing organisational structures combined with evolving professional roles that might influence nurse-led care. The complexities of these issues highlight the need to keep a focus on quality improvement, innovation and evidence-based practice as a central concern in the changing world of health care. The prevailing emphasis is on outcomes for patients, outcomes for health professionals and outcomes for the organisation. In charting our course it is vital that we make critical use of resources and organisational structures.

The topic of practice development has received a great of attention in the last few years, as approaches have rapidly evolved, hence the realistic synthesis of evidence relating to practice development put forward by McCormack et al. (2007). It would be very worthwhile to consider McCormack's findings and recommendations in the embryonic stage of setting up a nurse-led pre-admission clinic.

Quality improvement

Managing the costs and quality of patient outcomes continues to be a driving force in health care. Therefore, the quality improvement variable is concerned with benchmarking, audit and the measurement of practice against set standards. Throughout this chapter I have referred to different frameworks for understanding the nature of pre-operative assessment; for example, the pre-operative assessment programme (NHS Modernisation Agency 2004), attempts to standardise pre-operative testing produced by NICE (2003) with the emergence of specific guidelines and BADS (2006) directory of procedures, are all very useful for benchmarking purposes. The highest priority by far entails a firm focus on patients' experience of pre-assessment and to involve them closely in developing and defining outcome measure for developing a new service.

Continuous quality improvement, benchmarking and service re-engineering to drive policy directives are often shaped by a top-down corporate initiatives (Chin and Hamer 2006). However, if little attention is given to the valid knowledge and true expertise of practitioners in the practice environment, there is a danger that all those 'us-them' barriers will inhibit creativity. The commitment to changing the culture of care and birthing practice development is grounded in the convergence of corporate initiatives combined with team working. This empowers practitioners working at a clinical level to contribute innovative ideas and creative thinking in regard to meeting patient need (Chin and Hamer 2006). The existence of a more collaborative culture supports the implementation of organisational priorities with organic approaches to practice development.

Innovation and creativity

Innovation is concerned with 'doing things better and differently' (Hamer 2007). Policy documents are drenched in innovative ideas and have obvious application for day surgery. For instance, the NHS modernisation Agency highlighted that almost half a million in-patient beds could be available each year through improved methods of working. Expanding day surgery is number one in the '10 High Impact Changes' suggested as part of the NHS Modernisation Agenda (NHS Modernisation Agency 2004). Day surgery is further enthused by a white paper 'Our health, our care, our stay' (DH 2006b), portraying the government's plan for improving community care, in part by shifting resources from hospital to primary care. Day-case surgery in a primary care setting is one way to drive day surgery forward, meeting government targets and with many clinical benefits for the patient (Smith et al. 2006).

Setting up a nurse-led pre-assessment unit requires innovation. The journey requires the clinical team to provide creativity, clarity of purpose and focus (Chin and Hamer 2006), using a systematic and intentional way of working. One creative way forward is to utilise an organic approach that is symmetrical with practice development at an organisational level, creating a climate of enablement for team members, to explore innovative ideas, work through ambiguity and look at choices for action (Chin and Hamer 2006). Collective action is fundamental in influencing and driving the change process forward dynamically. The process can also be greatly enhanced by the accreditation programme (Totterdell 2004) and benchmarking can be set against the accreditation criteria (Box 3.4).

Evidence-Based Practice

The third vital ingredient that empowers practice development is EBP. The debate about what constitutes evidence-based practice is evolving. Clearly, quantitative evidence (chiefly from RCTs) has been the gold standard, the significant paradigm. Nevertheless, two differing perspectives on what constitutes evidence is emerging (Rycroft-Malone 2006). One view restricts evidence specifically to mean research findings and the other embraces a broader evidence base, including research findings, protocols, health practitioner's knowledge and patient expertise. Scott-Findlay and Pollock (2004) argue that experiential knowledge of the practitioner and patient experience are not powerful types of evidence, despite their influence. They go on to suggest that labelling them, as evidence is problematic because they are not valuable. The implications of such issues for clinical practice are noted by Rycroft-Malone (2006) including epistemology and ontology concerns regarding knowledge creation, perception and interpretation.

Despite epistemological concerns, health professionals attempting to facilitate practice development will need to embrace sound evidence. This will involve the interplay of factors and processes (Thompson 2003) that underpin EBP. The process is often complex because of competing interests, value conflicts and experiential knowledge among team members. However, different types of information influence the process, including protocols, research evidence, preference, and cultural and local contextual variables.

There is some striking evidence of successful intervention in pre-assessment cited throughout this chapter. For example, 'Best Practice' in the pre-admission care of patients (Pearson et al. 2004) pointed to two effective interventions, the first related to pre-operative telephone screening or questionnaire, and the second to a pre-admission appointment a few days prior to admission. Impressive results also revealed the usefulness of music and short stories to reduce pre-operative anxiety (Markland and Hardy 1993; Lee et al. 2004; Cooke et al. 2005), which is clearly useful for underpinning education on anxiety care.

Thus, the concept of practice development calls into play notion of robust interrelatedness, moving towards synthesis of quality improvement, innovation and EBP. The accreditation programme has four distinct pillars that includes those outlined in Box 3.4:

Box 3.4 Pillars of the Accreditation Programme *(© CDHPP, University of Leeds 2002)*

■ **Sustainable Practice Development**	Focusing on lasting achievements which can be sustained in real world environments
■ **Intentional Improvement**	Systematic planning
■ **Building Capacity for the Future**	Visible commitment to developing the resourcefulness of all team members
■ **Professional Accountability**	Recognising/valuing individual and collective responsibility

Accreditation

Any organisation that is concerned with quality improvement of patient-centred care and practice development will make it possible for those teams who are highly committed to gain accreditation. Several programmes are available for enabling clinical teams to gain nationally recognised accreditation in practice development, at university level (CDHPP 2007). If setting up a nurse-led pre-admission clinic is to become an established practice development initiative, it will probably involve the working group signing up to a practice development accreditation programme. The programme of study enables clinical teams to flourish in unique ways. In any working team there is probably a rich collection of abilities and interests, which could be drawn into remarkable ways of working if study days or workshops are undertaken. Above all else, creative facilitation styles, including leadership with the ability to involve users, invite a fresh approach to understanding the way forward.

The structured programme of study usually begins with a three-day residential course, offering an introduction to the accreditation process, including the exploration of leadership behaviours. This is followed by one-day workshops on a variety of themes, including, for example, 'innovation and creativity', 'systematic planning, prioritising and resource usage' and 'evaluation methods'. The content is not merely theoretical: it stimulates teams to subject their practice to reflection, with great attention being paid to the development loop. A crucial factor reported by Chin and Hamer (2006) is that the programme enables the participants to 'clarify their thinking', 'sharpen their focus' on the improvement initiative and 'recognise the potential of existing organisational strategies' to support the improvement work. It is vital to promote a climate that encourages practitioners to confront the realities of their practice development initiative, and in particular to assess patient outcomes.

The accreditation pathway

The accreditation process falls into two distinct stages. The first is awarded approximately one year following the start of the practice development initiative. At this juncture, firm evidence portraying that the working team is meeting the majority of the criteria outlined in Box 3.5 is required. Although practice development is tremendously appealing and offers a new expansiveness, new initiatives often evolves at a pace that matches organic approaches. Significantly, a heightened level of activity and growth are essential. The second stage is awarded in the region of two years following the enrolment date, on the condition that team evidence meets all the stipulated criteria to an optimal level. This implies that practice development is effective and fruitful. While the structure and format for accreditation might vary, the

Box 3.5 Accreditation criteria for practice development in a nurse-led pre-assessment unit © *CDHPP University of Leeds, 2007*

1. The pre-assessment unit has a clear and defined group of day surgery patients, which is reflected in the membership of the team.
2. The working team has chosen the accreditation approach itself.
3. The team has a shared vision for the practice development unit.
4. An approach to leadership is identified, which will facilitate the team in sustainable development, evaluation and dissemination of its work.
5. The unit has an explicit framework for organising and developing best practice, which incorporates devolved decision-making, staff and patient empowerment and partnership working.
6. Each team member is proactively involved in professional development, which is clearly related to patient-care need, and the plan for the development in the unit team as a whole.
7. The unit's development plan identifies the resources requirements needed in order to achieve accreditation in terms of time, expertise and financial support.
8. The unit's development plan includes the process for public and community engagement and disseminating evaluated practices both within the organisation and externally.
9. The unit team will have a reciprocal partnership with a centre of education, in order to support the development of clinical practice and theory.
10. The unit develops a rigorous, evidenced-based approach to practice.
11. The unit/team and the individuals within it are actively engaged in reflection and active learning.
12. The unit/team exhibits tangible evidence of creativity and innovation in relation to patient care issues and units developments.
13. Developments within the unit are evaluated and reviewed in terms of impact on patient, organisation and staff, and advises the broader senior management team.
14. The unit acts as an agent of change within the organisation, the region and nationally, publicising its success to promote the value of best practice.
15. The unit requires a steering group, which will focus, and coordinate the strategic direction of the unit.

key point is to recognise the richness of the ecology of accreditation. Evaluation is an important contributory factor to practice development and will be addressed in the following sections.

Evaluating services

Evaluation has an important function; it is a method of giving systematic feedback to working teams involved in innovative programmes such as setting up a nurse-led pre-admission clinic. If facilitated well, it can offer assurance and the data collected sheds light on the development loop. The findings and recommendations should be made available to the working group as a basis for discussion, in order that an action plan can be drawn up for further improvement in care. Ideally each evaluation process will generate such a plan, and the next round will provide data on whether the previous action plan has been effectively implemented. There is a great possibility of setting a virtuous cycle in motion, with huge outcomes in terms of effective patient care and job satisfaction.

There are a wide range of evaluation strategics than can be employed. Great discernment is needed in the selection process, because practice development units have diverse characteristics, and patient outcomes will relate to the work undertaken at a local level. Apart from variability, patient preparedness for day surgery is dependent on pre-assessment intervention which might influence, for example, the 'did attend' or 'did not attend rate', or anxiety management on the day of surgery itself. Evaluation of a pre-assessment practice development initiative is best integrated with the overall evaluation strategy for day surgery. Evaluating the quality of innovative nursing initiatives and care is indeed complex because it is influenced by dynamic factors such as professional structures (Rice et al. 2007), leadership styles, and the subtleties of the organisational culture and subcultures.

Approaches and frameworks

Evaluation methodologies can utilise quantitative or qualitative techniques. There is increasing evidence to suggest that multiple approaches, or, according to McCormack (2007), a strategic level of evaluation, are useful when attempting to create a robust, evaluative culture. McCormack goes on to suggest that a traditional approach to evaluation is not helpful, emphasising the need to develop a framework that is consistent with the practice development intervention. The pluralistic evaluation of practice development units was put forward by Gerrish (2001), pointing to seven categories:

Pluralistic Evaluation

1. Achieving optimum practice
2. Providing a patient-centred service
3. Disseminating innovative practice
4. Team working
5. Enabling practitioners to develop their full potential
6. Adopting a strategic approach to change
7. Autonomous functioning.

The criteria are based on feedback from stakeholders involved in six practice development units. However, they are not adequate because 'optimum practice' is not the gold standard and seems to be caught up in a contradiction, because the need is so intense to facilitate 'best practice' or 'excellence in practice'. Moreover, the outcome features of evaluation, especially in terms of patient benefits, are lacking (Gerrish 2001). Evaluation methods and tools for data collection have not been carefully considered. Perhaps a richer conception of evaluation is put forward by Rice et al. (2007), using an expert panel process.

Expert panel concept model

A more contemporary approach to the evaluation of nursing practice is the notion of expert peer review, which has been utilised successfully in the UK (Dugdall et al. 2004). Peer review relies on judgements by expert professionals to evaluate the quality of nursing care. The account of the quality framework formulated by Rice et al. (2007:95) is indeed attractive, as 'being cyclical in nature and designed to evolve to meet the needs of patients, nurses and other stakeholders'. Understandably, the central features of this model relate to the task of evaluating patient care and promoting excellence in patient care. The main aspirations of the evaluation are to: evaluate practice standards, address problems, promote and share clinical innovations, and promote better patient outcomes. Non-surprisingly, the expert panel explore the suitability of this approach with potential clinical professionals.

A multi-method approach to data collection is advocated by Rice et al. (2007: 97). They go on to suggest that tool design should be based on 'best practice', organisational policy, practice guidelines and expert knowledge. A pilot programme of the expert panel approach to test the process and data collection tools was recently undertaken in Australia (Rice et al. 2007). The schedule involved eight wards with several modes of care delivery including day surgery. Tools employed for data collection included survey questionnaires, focus groups and clinical audits. Additionally, 'a structured speciality presentation involving strict assessment criteria was given by the ward or unit undergoing evaluation to show their clinical innovation'. The

Table 3.1 Evaluation framework

General Evaluation Areas	Speciality Practice Areas Evaluated
Patient preparedness for day procedure	Model of care
Respiratory care	Redevelopment of the endoscopy service
Pain management	Commissioning of day surgery
Medication administration	Development of day medical service
Documentation	
Medical emergency practice	
Staff professional development	
Communication	
Rostering and resource allocation	
Performance management	

evaluation framework required some modification for day surgery: evaluating both general and speciality practice includes for example, areas outlined in Table 3.1.

Overall, the expert panel process was very effective in the evaluation of day surgery care, recognising achievement of best practice and making recommendations for improvement in some areas. Although this approach is not directly transferable to day surgery units in the UK, its principals are generalisable. This significant framework brings into focus the uniqueness of evaluating day surgery care with excellent potential for evaluating practice development. However, some of the general evaluation areas have a kind of 'biomedical' orientation. This could be modified and sharpened, designing both general and speciality evaluation areas and audit tools to fit the idiosyncratic nature of any day surgery context.

Tool for evaluating a one stop pre-assessment service

There seems to be a range of new validated tools emerging that could possibly be employed for evaluating pre-assessment intervention. For example, a new tool has been developed and validated (Karthikeyan et al. 2007) for measuring patient satisfaction with a one stop cataract pre-assessment service, where surgery is performed at the second visit. The validated questionnaire appears to be useful in evaluating the pre-assessment intervention in conjunction with the day of surgery itself. This particular tool could be modified and utilised by other cataract service providers, especially those involved in developing new initiatives to improve access. This, however, is only a partial answer. It would not satisfy those with an interest in evaluating health professional's perceptions or the benefits to the organisation in terms of streamlining services. The central point is that multi-forms of evaluation might be justifiable, hence the significance of the strategic framework suggested by McCormack et al. (2007).

Conclusion

This chapter has travelled a long way, starting with an exploration of the emergence of nurse-led interventions and moving on to nurse-led pre-admission clinics. The evolvement of nurse-led interventions was initially perceived as utilising nurses to help doctors with their activities, increase cost effectiveness and in response to the government pushing the modernisation agenda. Although the ontology of nursing has lost ground in the construction of new roles, there are definitely many benefits for patients. Nurses currently facilitate credible nurse-led pre-admission clinics, and 'one stop shops' which increases access to day surgery services. They offer a rich and dynamic range of services such as holistic assessment of fitness for day surgery, undertake extended roles, educate patients and their carers, explore lifestyle management and facilitate health promotion. As the 21st century unfolds, the expansion of day surgery on a widespread scale stimulates the search for more robust clinical effectiveness and for an economic process far better than we have at present. This positive expansion poses creative challenges for those involved in developing nurse-led services.

Nurses who desire autonomy and are willing and able to undertake practice development initiatives in setting up a nurse-led pre-assessment clinic, need to address important considerations. This strategic task requires energetic, optimistic, highly motivated and enthusiastic team players that are strongly committed to the vision of the new service. The prevailing emphasis is on rich patient outcomes, grounded in policy drivers and underpinned by evidence-based practice and innovation. Ideally, it should both be tackled at a local level and integrated with organisational strategies. This means that it is essential to have new nurse-led services symmetrical with organisational goals to properly address strategic planning and expansiveness. A new service requires careful evaluation in terms of offering systematic feedback to the innovative team involved. Drawing on a multi-method approach is vital to ensure that patient perceptions, health professional perceptions and organisational perceptions are examined thoroughly. The expert panel approach has a great capacity for evaluating practice development, highlighting clinical excellence, deficits in care and providing recommendations.

References

Bramhall, J. (2002) The role of nurses in pre-operative assessment. *Nursing Times*, 98 (40), 34–5.

Boyle, J.S. and Andrews, M.M. (2003) Andrews/Boyle assessment guide. In: *Transcultural Concepts in Nursing Care*, (eds M.M. Andrews and J.S. Boyle), 4th ed. pp. 533–9. Lippincott Williams and Wilkins, Philadelphia.

British Association of Day Surgery (2006) *BADS Directory of Procedures*. British Association of Day Surgery, London.

Centre for the Development of Healthcare Policy and Practice (2007) *Practice Development Programme*, School of Healthcare, University of Leeds. http://www.cdhpp.leeds.ac.uk (accessed 24 August 2008)

Chang, B. (1980) Evaluation of health care professional in facilitating self-care: Review of the literature and a conceptual model. *Advances in Nursing Science*, 3 (1), 43–58.

Chin, H. and Hamer, S. (2006). Enabling practice development: Evaluation of a pilot programme to effect integrated and organic approaches to practice development. *Practice Development Health Care*, 5 (3), 126–44.

Clark, K., Voase R., Cato, G., Fletcher, I.R. and Thomson, P.J. (2000) Patients' experience of day case surgery: Feedback from a nurse-led pre-admission clinic. *Ambulatory Surgery*, 8, 93–6.

Conner, M. and Norman, P. (2005) *Predicting Health Behaviour*, 2nd ed. Open University Press, Maidenhead, England.

Connolly, D. (2003) State of the art: Orthopaedic anaesthesia. *Anaesthesia*, 58 (12), 1189–93.

Cooke T., Fitzpatrick R. and Smith I. (2004) *Achieving Day Surgery Targets: A practical approach towards achieving efficiency in day case units in the United Kingdom*. Advanced Medical Publications, London.

Cooke, M., Chaboyer, W., Schluter, P. and Hiratos, M. (2005) The effect of music on preoperative anxiety in day surgery. *Journal of Advanced Nursing*, 52 (1), 47–55.

Cortina, M. and Marrone, M. (2003) *Attachment theory and the Psychoanalytic Process*. Whurr, London.

Coyler, H.M. (2004) The construction and development of health professionals: Where will it end? *Journal of Advanced Nursing*, 48 (4), 406–12.

Craig, S.E. (2005) Does nurse-led pre-operative assessment reduce the cancellation rate of elective surgical in-patient procedures? A systematic review of the research literature. *British Journal of Anaesthetic and Recovery Nursing*, 6 (3), 41–7.

Department of Health NHS Modernisation Agency (2004) *10 High Impact Changes for Service Improvement and Delivery*. http://wise.nhs.uk/cmsWise/HIC/HIC+Intro.htm (accessed 24 November 2007).

Department of Health (1999a) *Agenda for Change: Modernising the NHS Pay System*. The Stationery Office, London.

Department of Health (1999b) *Making a Difference: Strengthening the Nursing, Midwifery and Health Visitor Contribution to Health and Health Care*. The Stationery Office, London.

Department of Health (2000) *The NHS Plan: Creating a 21st Century NHS*. HMSO, London.

Department of Health (2006a) *National Target and Policy Initiatives*. www.dh.gov.uk/reducingmrsa (accessed 21 December 2007).

Department of Health (2006b) http://www.dh.gov.uk/Policy and Guidance/Organisation Policy/ (accessed 28 December 2007)

Department of Health (2007) *Definitions of Overweight and Obesity*. http://www.dh/gov.uk (accessed 27 December 2007)

Dugdall, H., Lamb, C. and Carlisle A. (2004) Improving quality care through a nursing review team. *Clinical Governance: An International Journal*, 9 (3), 155–61.

Feinstein, D., Eden, D. and Craig, G. (2005) *The Healing Power of EFT and Energy Psychology*. Piakus, London.

Friedman, Z., Wong, D.T. and Chung, F. (2003) What are the ambulatory surgical patient selection criteria in Canada? (Abstract). *Canadian Journal of Anaesthesia*, 50 (suppl.), A16.

Gardener, G., Chang, A. and Suffield, C. (2006) Making nursing work: Breaking through the role confusion of advanced nursing practice. *Journal of Advanced Nursing*, 57 (4), 382–91.

Gerrish, K. (2001) A Pluralistic evaluation of nursing/practice development units. *Journal of Clinical Nursing*, 10 (1), 109–18.

Gilmartin, J. (2004) Day surgery: Patients' perceptions of nurse-led pre-admissions clinic. *Journal of Clinical Nursing*, 13, 243–50.

Gilmartin, J. (2007) Contemporary day surgery: Patients' experience of discharge and recovery. *Journal of Clinical Nursing*, 16, 1109–17.

Gilmartin, J. and Wright, K. (2007) The nurse's role in day surgery: A literature review. *International Nursing Review*, 54 (2), 183–90.

Grypdonck, M.H.F. (2006) Qualitative Health Research in the Era of Evidence-based practice. *Qualitative Health Research*, 16 (10), 1371–85.

Hamer, S. (2007) Doing things better and differently. *Practice Development Health Care*, 6 (3), 176.

Jackson, I. (2007) Day surgery overview: Where are we now, how did we get here and where are we going? *Current Anaesthesia and Critical Care*, 18, 176–80.

Jiménez, A., Artigas C., Elia, M., Casamayar, C., Gracia, J.A. and Martínez M. (2006) Cancellations in ambulatory day surgery: Ten years observational study *Ambulatory Surgery* 12 (3), 119–23.

Karthikeyan, M., Dahlmann-Noor, A.H., Gupta, N. and Vivian, A.J. (2007) Development and validation of a new tool to assess patient satisfaction with cataract services. *Clinical Governance: An International Journal*, 12 (4), 249–59.

Kerr, J., Weitkunat, R. and Moretti, M. (2005) *ABC of Behaviour Change: A Guide to Successful Disease Prevention and Health Promotion*. Elsevier Churchill Livingstone, London.

Kinley, H., Czoski-Murray, C., George, S., McCabe, C., Primose, J., Reilly, C., Wood, R., Nicholson, P., Healey, C., Read, S., Norman, J., Janke, E., Alhameed, H., Fernandes, N. and Thomas, E. (2002) Effectiveness of appropriately trained nurses in preoperative assessment: Randomised controlled equivalence/non-inferior trial. *British Medical Journal*, 325, 1–5.

Korp, P. (2005) Health on the Internet: Implications for health promotion. *Health Education Research*, 21 (1), 78–86.

Lee, D., Henderson, A. and Shum, D. (2004) The effects of music on preprocedure anxiety in Hong Kong Chinese day patients. *Journal of Clinical Nursing*, 13, 297–303.

Lloyd-Jones, M. (2005) Role development and effective practice in specialist and advanced practice roles in acute hospital settings: Systematic review and meta-synthesis. *Journal of Advanced Nursing*, 49 (2), 191–209.

Markland, D. and Hardy, L. (1993) Anxiety, relaxation and anaesthesia for day case surgery. *British Journal of Clinical Psychology*, 32, 493–504.

Marsden, J. and Shaw, M.E. (2007) The development of advanced practice roles in ophthalmic nursing. *Practice Development for Health Care*, 6 (2), 119–30.

McCabe, C. and Timmins, F. (2006) *Communication Skills for Nursing Practice.* Palgrave Macmillan, London.

MacCormack, B., Wright, J., Dewer, B. and Harvey, G. (2007) A realistic synthesis of evidence relating to practice development – methodology and methods. *Practice Development for Health Care*, 6 (1), 5–24.

MacCormack, B., Wright, J., Dewer, B. and Harvey, G. (2007) A realistic synthesis of evidence relating to practice development – findings from the literature analysis. *Practice Development for Health Care*, 6 (1), 25–58.

MacCormack, B., Wright, J., Dewer, B. and Harvey, G. (2007) A realistic synthesis of evidence relating to practice development – recommendations. *Practice Development for Health Care*, 6 (1), 76–80.

Macdonald, M. and Bodzak, W. (1999) The performance of self-managing day surgery nurse team. *Journal of Advanced Nursing*, 29 (4), 859–68.

Mitchell, M.J. (2000b) Anxiety management: A distinct nursing role in day surgery. *Ambulatory Surgery* (8), 119–27.

Mitchell, M.J. (2005) *Anxiety Management in Adult Day Surgery: A Nursing Perspective.* Whurr, London.

Mitchell, M.J. (2006) Nursing knowledge and the expansion of day surgery in the United Kingdom. *Ambulatory Surgery*, 12 (3), 125–30.

Muir Gray, J.A. (2001) *Evidence-Based Healthcare*, 2nd edn. Churchill Livingstone, Edinburgh.

National Health Service Management Executive (1991) *Junior Doctors: The New Deal.* HMSO, London.

National Health Service Management Executive (1993) *Report by the Day Surgery Task Force.* HMSO, London.

National Health Service Modernisation Agency (2002) *National Good Practice Guidelines on Pre-operative Assessment for Day Surgery.* HMSO, London.

National Health Service Modernisation Agency (2004) *10 High Impact Changes for Service Improvement and Delivery.* HMSO, London.

National Institute for Clinical Excellence (2003) *Pre-operative Tests: The Use of Routine Pre-operative Tests for Elective Surgery.* www.nice.org.uk.

Orem, D.E. (1971, 1980, 1985, 1995, 2001) *Nursing: Concepts of Practice*, 1st, 2nd, 3rd, 4th, 5th & 6th edn. Mosby, London.

O'Shea, M. (2007) Hospital can be child's play. Pre-admission visits to prepare children for day surgery are proving effective in Cork. *World of Irish Nursing*, 15, 2.

Page, S. (2002) The role of practice development in modernising the NHS. *Nursing Times*, 98, 11.

Page, S. and Hamer, S. (2002) Practice development – time to realize the potential. *Practice Development in Health Care*, 1, 2–17.

Pearson, A., Richardson, M. and Cairns, M. (2004) 'Best practice' in day surgery units: A review of the evidence. *Journal of Ambulatory Surgery*, 11, 49–54.

Read, S. and Robert-Davis, M. (2000) *Preparing Nurse Practitioners for the 21st Century. Executive summary from the Report of the Project Realising Specialist and Advanced Nursing Practice: Establishing the parameters of and identifying the competence for nurse practitioner roles and evaluating programmes of preparation.* Sheffield University, Sheffield.

Rhodes, L., Miles, G. and Pearson A. (2006) Patient subjective experience and satisfaction during the perioperative period in day surgery: A systematic review. *International Journal of Nursing Practice*, 12, 178–92.

Rice, S.M., Van Slobe, A. and Rathgeber, D. (2007) Nursing practice evaluation using an expert panel process. *Clinical Governance: An International Journal*, 12 (2), 93–101.

Richardson, G. and Maynard, A. (1995) *Fewer doctors? More nurses? A review of the knowledge base of doctor-nurse substitution*, discussion paper 135. Centre for Health Economics/York Health Economics Consortium/NHS Centre for Reviews and Dissemination, University of York, York.

Rogan, F. and Timmins, F. (2004) Improving communication in day surgery settings. *Nursing Standard*, 19 (7), 37–42.

Rogers, C.A. (1980) *A Way of Being*. Houghton Mifflin, Boston.

Royal College of Nursing (2002) *Nurse Practitioner: An RCN Guide to the Nurse Practitioner Role, Competencies and Programme Accreditation*. RCN, London.

Royal College of Surgeons of England (1992) *Commission on the provision of surgical services: Guidelines for day case surgery*. HMSO, London.

Rycroft-Malone, J. (2006) The politics of the evidence-based practice movements. *Journal of Research in Nursing*, 11 (2), 95–108.

Scott, A. (2001) How much information is too much information for patients? *Journal of Integrated Care Pathways*, 5, 119–25.

Scott-Findlay, S. and Pollock, C. (2004) Evidence, research, knowledge: A call for conceptual clarity. *Worldviews on Evidence-Based Nursing*, 1, (2), 92–7.

Shah. J. and Sill, S. (2007) Evaluation of information leaflets for flexible cystoscopy. *Clinical Governance*, 12 (1), 38–41.

Smith, I., Cooke, T., Jackson, I. and Fitzpatrick, R. (2006) Rising to the challenges of achieving day surgery targets. *Anaesthesia*, 61 (12), 1191–9.

Smith, I. (2007) Day surgery for all: Updated selection criteria. *Current Anaesthesia and Critical Care*, 18, 181–7.

Stern, D. (1985) *The Interpersonal World of the Infant: A view from Psychoanalysis and Developmental Psychology*. Basic Books, New York.

Thompson, C. and Dowding, D. (2002) *Clinical Decision Making and Judgement in Nursing*. Churchill Livingstone, Edinburgh, London.

Thompson, C. (2003) Clinical experience as evidence in evidence-based practice. *Journal of Advanced Nursing*, 43, (3), 230–7.

Thompson, C., Cullum, N., McCaughton, D., Sheldon, T. and Raynor, P. (2004) Nurses, information use, and clinical decision making: The real world potential for evidence-based decision in nursing. *British Medical Journal*, 7, 68–72.

Totterdell, B. (2004) The practice development accreditation programme at the University of Leeds. *Practice Development in Health Care*, 3 (3), 130–42.

Walgrove, H. (2004) Piloting a nurse-led gynaecology pre-operative assessment clinic, *Nursing Times*, 100 (3), 38–41.

Williams, A., Ching, M. and Loader, J. (2003) Assessing patient satisfaction with day surgery at a metropolitan public hospital. *Australian Journal of Advanced Nursing*, 21 (1), 35–4.

Practice Development

Robert McSherry, Kay Scott and Sharon Farlow

Introduction

This chapter introduces practice development and how to apply practice development initiatives in the day surgery unit. The emphasis of the chapter is on how nurses can utilise these initiatives in enhancing the care and services offered in the quest for quality in day surgery services. The chapter will also offer practical ways to evaluate practice development initiatives in day surgery.

Background

Day Surgery is defined as 'the admission of selected patients to hospital for a planned surgical procedure, returning home on the same day. 'True day surgery' patients are day case patients who require full operating theatre facilitates/and or general anaesthetic.' (DH 2002:2).

The DH (2002) further suggests that procedures performed in outpatient departments and endoscopy units are not included within the definition of day surgery. The Audit Commission however suggests that these categories can be labelled as 'Minor day case' (Audit Commission 2001) yet Jackson (2007:2) states that what 'many clinicians do not understand is that the Department of Health will only count a patient as a day case if they were placed on the waiting list for management as a day case by their surgeon; this is called their management intent.'

The Royal College of Surgeons (1992) reported that day surgery was the best option for 50% of patients undergoing elective procedures. However, performance across the United Kingdom was deemed by the Healthcare Commission as poor (HC 2005). This is in spite of the fact that in 1989, following the formation of British Association of Day Surgery (BADS), emphasis was placed on safety, quality and excellence through enhancing practice.

Practice Development (PD) has recently been defined as

> . . . a continuous process of developing person-centred cultures. It is enabled by facilitators who authentically engage with individuals and teams to blend personal qualities and creative imagination with practice skills and practice wisdom. The learning that occurs brings about transformations of individual and team practices. This is sustained by embedding both processes and out-comes in corporate strategy. (Manley et al. 2008; Foundation of Nursing Studies online 2008).

McCormack et al. (2008) definition suggests that PD is ideal for promot-ing innovation and change with the Day Surgery Unit (DSU) because it advocates the need for collaboration, partnerships and team working. According to McSherry and Warr (2008), the drivers for innovation and changing through practice development within the day surgery unit arise from a combination of societal, political and professional factors such as those outlined in Box 4.1.

Box 4.1   *Drivers for practice development and quality in day surgery unit*

- rising patient/client, carer expectation
- increased dependency of those accessing services
- technological advances
- demographic changes in society
- changes in care delivery systems
- lack of public confidence in health care services
- threat of litigation
- demands for greater access to information.

To address and respond to the growing pressures to change, reform or modernise to keep up with the times, it is important that professionals working in day surgery recognise what, why and how practice development may aid the pursuit of excellence. For this to happen it is imperative that we understand what we mean by the term 'practice development'.

What do we mean by practice development?

Activity 4.1

Reflective Question

Write down what you understand by the terms practice development

Read on and compare your notes with the remainder of the section.

Practice development is an approach that recognises the realities of external influence whilst allowing an individual service to focus on developing excellence in practice in all areas. It is an inclusive, 'bottom-up' approach to review and change the whole service, which puts the patient at the centre of the care process. It has many definitions (Kitson 1994; Bassett 1996; McCormack et al. 1999, 2008; Clarke and Wilcockson 2001; McSherry and Bassett 2002; Page and Hamer 2002; Garbett and McCormack 2001; Hynes 2004; McSherry and Warr 2006, 2008) which emphasise different aspects of these qualities. One we have found useful and applicable for practical delivery in day surgery is that offered by McSherry and Warr (2006): 'practice development's primary principles are centred on promoting patient-centeredness through the utilisation of a facilitative approach to team working, collaboration and partnership building'.

The facilitative approach to innovation and change offers an ideal vehicle to utilise targets and standards through an inclusive and empowering way to develop local practice making PD applicable to the day surgery settings. Within the context of day surgery, PD is about encouraging individuals, teams and organisations to improve practice through innovation and change (McSherry and Bassett 2002). Practice development plays a pivotal role in fostering a culture and context that nurtures evidence-based nursing. This, according to Page and Hamer (2002:6), is because PD centrally focuses on activities which enhance the culture, working environment and journey of care by promoting person-centred quality improvement(s) through encouraging individuals, teams and organisations to innovate and change using an evidence base.

Similarly PD is appropriate for professionals working in day surgery because it happens within the professional's 'own' practice setting and is about the enhancement and growth of personal, professional and/or organisational standards and quality of services by involving and focusing on the patients and clients specific needs. Excellence in day surgery units as suggested by McSherry (2004) requires team-working, interdisciplinary collaboration, effective communication, internal and external partnerships and a willingness to learn and share with and from each other – including users of the service. You will notice from other chapters in this book, particularly chapters 4, 5, 6 and 7, that these practices are essential in all aspects of day surgery in providing high quality care that is patient-centred. Professionals working in day surgery units need to recognise and embrace the value of PD as an integral part of their roles and take responsibility to advance and evaluate practice using the key principals, characteristics and values of PD. So what are the key characteristics' and qualities of PD for day surgery units?

Characteristics and qualities required to take practice development forward in day surgery

A description of the characteristics, qualities and skills in practice development based on McCormack and Garbett (2003), outlined in Table 4.1, indicates that the characteristics and qualities of practice developers include the abilities to encourage and motivate staff to innovate and/or evaluate practices in the quest for improved quality. Successful PD is dependent upon advancing and supporting individuals to develop certain essential skills and attributes so that they can progress and or evaluate practice as part of the change processes.

Table 4.1 A description of the characteristics, qualities and skills in PD (*adapted from McCormack & Garbett 2003; McSherry and Driscoll 2004*)

Characteristics	Qualities	Skills	Individual personal attributes
■ promoting and facilitating change ■ translation and communication ■ responding to external influences ■ education ■ audit, quality and evaluation	■ affection ■ having vision ■ motivation ■ empathy ■ experiential ■ can motivate ■ respect ■ experience ■ approachable ■ agent of change ■ supportive ■ good listener	■ cognitive ■ political awareness ■ communicative ■ facilitative ■ clinical	ability to: ■ motivate ■ facilitate ■ innovate ■ inform ■ encourage ■ support

Table 4.1 highlights the essential characteristics, qualities, skills and personal attributes which can contribute in making PD occur in the day surgery unit. Some day surgery units are now introducing facilitators, advisers or developers to support and facilitate change. However, giving the opportunity for individuals and teams to take responsibility for advancing and evaluating their own or teams practice as part of ever changing agenda, is not the case in many day surgery units. McSherry and Warr (2008) recommend the implementation of an identified practice developer to support organisations and teams in enhancing quality within busy, stressful and time-pressured day surgery units. Several models have been reported and commented upon which could be used as exemplars in developing PD within the day surgery unit (Glover 1998). Yet McSherry and Warr (2008) and Garbett and McCormack (2001) air caution when introducing PD so that the key roles and responsibilities are not tied in with other aspects of the governance agenda, because this makes the posts too big and difficult to operationalise successfully. It could be fair to suggest that to advance and evaluate practice within the day surgery unit, all professionals should possess the skills outlined in Table 4.1. The challenge for professionals in day surgery is in applying PD into practice.

Applying practice development initiatives in day surgery units

Hoban (2007) indicates that PD could be regarded as a 'macrosystem' for enhancing quality within a Health and Social Care Service and/or Trust. This is because PD can only occur with support and backing from organisational leaders and managers. However, Mohr et al. (2004) argue that 'macrosystems' are comprised of 'microsystems' from within the organisation whose loyalty is first and foremost to their patients. Mohr et al. (2004) suggest that ultimately the outcomes of macrosystems can be no better than those of the microsystems from which they are formed. The idea of microsystems and macrosystems is a good analogy for viewing PD-based activities within the day surgery unit, which could be portrayed as a microsystem stemming from the larger organisational structures. Put simply, the recognition of a day surgery unit as a microsystem permits a structured approach to enhancing PD activities and implementing PD initiatives on a relatively small scale. This acknowledgement can be used to promote awareness of PD in day surgery as an essential mechanism to enhance the objectives of the microsytem (organisation), alongside other microsystems within the macrosystem.

The challenge facing individuals and teams working with day surgery units is to continuously scrutinise their practices in the quest for quality. Bates (2000) emphasises that an innovative approach to care is necessary and that members of the multidisciplinary team need to work together, possibly crossing boundaries. Bates (2000) further reiterates the fostering and dissemination of research and change whilst being receptive to implementing ideas and changes that occur outside its boundaries. Practice development is ideal in fostering a shared vision through multi-disciplinary team working, because 'PD draws on many different and diverse disciplines, which in turn enables all professional functions to be integrated for the benefit of patients. It is a prerequisite to clinical effectiveness, continuous quality improvement and the development of a culture that facilitates the responsive and proactive action necessary for effective health care.' (Manley and McCormack 2003:23)

Taking Manley and McCormack's (2003) work into account and applying this to the day surgery unit setting, it is important to remember that for a successful innovation and change outcome the whole team are informed and involved at an appropriate level. Meaden and Solley (2003), as highlighted in Figure 4.1, outline possible members of the day surgery team and show the need to incorporate a diverse number of individuals when considering innovation and change through PD. A review of Figure 4.1 illustrates the importance of identifying team members in order to determine their roles, responsibilities and functions within identified PD systems and processes.

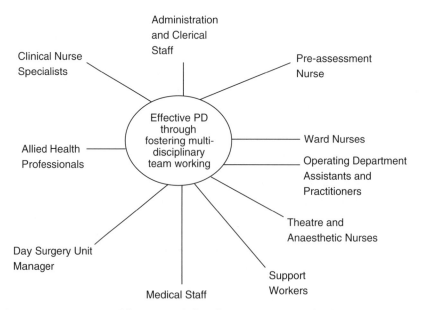

Figure 4.1 Promoting and fostering multidisciplinary team practice development within Day Surgery Units

Activity 4.2

Reflective Question

If you were about to instigate a change in practice, identify the team members and outline their potential involvement and impact of the change.

Read on and compare your notes with the remainder of the section.

Through Activity 4.2, you will have identified the importance of involving within the change process the majority of team members, similar to those identified in Figure 4.1. This process is essential in order to encourage multidisciplinary teamworking through collaboration and partnership building. The process of identifying and engaging team members enables the identification of leaders, managers and colleagues key to securing the right level of support, and in securing appropriate resources, for example financial backing. Furthermore, identifying team members highlights the necessity to engage and inform all team members (where possible and practical) on a regular basis. This ensures effective communication, continuity in the change process and an outcome of quality patient care.

Having identified the importance of sharing and communicating your vision and the need to adopt and multidisciplinary approach to collaboration and partnership building, the next stage to successful innovation and change is the development of a robust implementation and evaluation framework.

The Health Service Executive South, Nursing and Midwifery Planning Unit *A Strategy For Practice Development* (2006) offers an excellent chapter illustrating key systems and processes required to aid successful innovation and change. Table 4.2 has been adapted from this chapter and illustrates a logical and systematic series of phases deemed important when embarking on innovation and change in a day surgery unit.

For day surgery units to benefit from engaging with Table 4.2, it is essential that individuals and teams can identify and prioritise changes required in practice which may be in keeping with political, professional and local priorities. By following the sequence of phases identified in Table 4.2, innovation and change may be targeted to support PD within individual day surgery unit. Innovation and change, as illustrated in Table 4.2, is highly complex and challenging but significantly rewarding. In order to progress innovation and change in day surgery units efficiently and effectively, it is important to consider the following key areas: identification; challenges; evaluation and implementation of innovation and change.

Table 4.2 Adopting a structured approach to practice development in day surgery units

Phase	Key steps	Relevant to changing practice in DSU
	Identification of innovation and change	
Consider area for development	■ Indentify area ■ Detail issue of development ■ Describe current practice	Allows identification and rationale for change. Could be based on findings from incident reports/complaints, audits, research and patient/staff feedback.
Potential change required	■ Determine impetus ■ Consider barriers/conditions to change ■ Identify challenges	Imperative to highlight why the change is required and what conditions may facilitate this in reality.
	Challenges for innovation and change	
Stakeholders involved	■ Identify key stakeholder ■ Stakeholder analysis	Opinions and values are obtained from the outset which can inform and affect the change.
Working group	■ Recruit into group(s) ■ Identify roles and responsibilities ■ Establish terms of reference for group(s)	Essential for highlighting key individual roles and responsibilities in executing change. A minimum of two and a maximum of eight individuals are deemed important for a achieving a functional groups.
Practice setting	■ Context ■ Culture ■ Facilitation ■ Resources ■ Review existing evidence	Awareness and understating of organisational cultures and contexts are imperative factors affecting change. Skilled facilitation and resource allocation are key components of successful change.
	Implementation of innovation and change	
Action plan	■ Identify and set objectives ■ State how objectives to be achieved ■ Agree realist timeframe ■ Consensus agree ■ Gantt chart	A template highlighting key objectives and time frames is important in communicating the change processes.
Implementation	■ Prepare ■ Educate ■ Action	A critical stage where support and encouragement should be readily available to reduce resistance. A facilitative leadership style needs to be employed in order to engage and encourage participation.

Evaluation of innovation and change
Imperative in demonstrating the impact of change in and on practice.

Identification of innovation and change

According to McCormack et al. (2008), McSherry and Warr (2008), O'Neal and Manley (2007), Hoban (2007) and The Health Service Executive South, Nursing and Midwifery Planning Unit (2006), prior to embarking on any innovation and change, it is imperative to consider the area for development and why this important in enhancing patient-centred care. Enhancing patient-centred care within the day surgery unit according to Lewis et al. (2000) and JBI (2003) could focus on areas such as the following practices and or services which affect prolonged stays within the day surgery unit:

- **Pre-admission care** – assessments, investigations, telephone advice and screening.
- **Post admission care** – management of nausea and vomiting, pain control, burden on families.
- **Skill mix** – ensuring staffing and workloads are appropriate in meeting the vision, gaols and beliefs of the DSU.
- **Communications** – ensuring efficient and effective channels of communication are available for staff and patients.

Like Lewis et al. (2000) and JBI (2003), The Healthcare Commission (HC) (2005) have additionally identified areas in which day surgery practice could be developed in day surgery units and compare perceived current practices alongside recommendations for good practice Table 4.3.

The above examples are not exhaustive but can be used as a guide to stimulate PD within a day surgery unit. Having identified the area for innovation and change it is important that the various team members are actively encouraged to become involved with and take ownership of the change and associated processes.

Challenges for innovation and change

Following the identification of the innovation and change area, the next stage is to analyse the potential challenges and barriers which could impact on the change process. McSherry and Warr (2008) suggest that there are a myriad of individual and organisational tools and techniques available to support the change process in determining the potential challenges and barriers. Table 4.4 offers some examples of such tools and techniques.

The utilisation of assessment tools (such as those identified in Table 4.4) within the context of PD in day surgery can promote effective collaboration by identifying and resolving

Table 4.3 Potential areas for practice development (*adapted from Healthcare Commission 2005*)

	What happens	Good practice
Referral and booking	Referred to outpatients or clinic	Locally agreed referral criteria
		Referral designed to clarify special needs – assessment accounts for these in relation to planning surgical procedure
	Decision to admit	Options discussed with time to consider before consenting
		Information regarding whole procedure should be sufficient to allow informed choice and allay concerns
	Mutually convenient admission date and time offered and agreed	Arrival times staggered to minimise waits
		HC (2005) reported that admissions only partially booked with broad agreements.
Pre-admission	Given written information	Written information should include
		What to expect:
		■ Description of procedure
		■ Sequence of events
		■ Discharge
		Who to contact:
		■ For advice and help
		■ If they have a complaint
		May be re-assessed or telephoned if admission to be more than six weeks after initial assessment to avoid cancellations
On the day	Anaesthetic assessment confirmed	Facilities permit patients to undress, wait and be assessed in private
	Anaesthetic administered, operation or procedure performed	Optimally, in a dedicated day surgery theatre within the unit
	Recovery completed on bed/trolley/ reclining chair in day surgery unit or ward	Check for excessive pain or complications before discharge
		Adult patients discharged by nurses/non-medical staff in accordance with protocol
On and after discharge	Given written discharge, treatment given	This should include
		■ Post-discharge medication
		■ Aftercare required
		■ Dedicated phone number
		If there are any concerns the patient should be telephoned at home within 24 hours of discharge

- *Organisational issues:* Implementing a new service or reviewing and redesigning existing services
- *Conflicting expectations:* To review conflicts of interest between professional groups, teams and individuals.
- *Communication issues;* with, between and within individual teams and the organisation.
- *Cultural differences;* between services and departments.
- *Resource availability:* for existing or planned service developments.

Table 4.4 Tools and techniques to aid practice development in day surgery unit (*adapted from McSherry and Warr 2008*)

Force Field Analysis (FFA)

A structured group analysis technique that attempts to maximise the success of a proposed solution. When you have agreed on a solution to a problem you may well find the technique useful.

Force Field Analysis is a way of identifying the forces and factors in place that support or work against your solution. You may then be able to develop some further ideas to reinforce the driving forces and reduce or eliminate the restraining forces.

Political, Economical Social and Technological Assessment (PEST analysis)

An organisation's operating environment can be analysed by looking at:

- External forces (*those factors that an organisation has no control over*)
- Internal forces (*factors that an organisation has direct control over*)

The external environment of an organisation can be analysed by conducting a **PEST** analysis. This is a simple analysis of an organisation's **P**olitical, **E**conomical **S**ocial and **T**echnological environment.

Strengths, Weaknesses, Opportunities and Threats (SWOT Analysis)

SWOT analysis is commonly used in marketing as a tool to define plans and set strategies. The term **SWOT** analysis is about the identification of **S**trengths, **W**eaknesses, **O**pportunities and **T**hreats; it can help define what needs to be done to adapt to new roles.

SWAINE analysis

A self-evaluation technique that allows individuals to identify their personal development needs. The key meaning of SWAIN is **S**trengths, **W**eaknesses, **A**spirations, **I**nterests and **N**eeds. Following the self-evaluation an individual action plan can be established for moving forward.

Values Clarification Exercise

This is a tool frequently used within practice development (Manley 1997) for 'developing a common shared vision and purpose. It can be used for developing a common vision about areas as different as development of role definitions, competency, or curriculum frameworks, to, developing strategic direction for different purposes' (RCN 2002:1).

The benefits of such approaches according to McSherry and Johnson (2005) could be improved quality, enhanced communication, shared working an understanding of complementary points of view and enhanced productivity/outcomes. The challenge facing those who wish to develop practice within the day surgery unit is identifying, from the available tools and techniques, those that are most appropriate in supporting the process and also determining the effectiveness of the change. This is imperative to enable others to learn and share from the experience and avoid constantly reinventing the wheel. Even the smallest of tools and techniques require time, investment and resourcing to be useful. McPhail (1997) suggests several factors that may impede the process of change, including: reluctance to move from a safe situation; poor planning; inability to share the vision; lack of communication; and inadequate resourcing. Having identified the challenges surrounding innovation and change in practice, it is imperative to establish ways and means of implementing innovation and change in practice.

Implementation of innovation and change

In the initial stage of the change process, it is essential to identify resources in the form of personnel, including facilitators of change.

McSherry and Warr (2008) argue that facilitation is an important factor for effective PD. Facilitation according to Collins (1987) is defined as 'to make easy or easier'. Facilitation within the context of PD is about understanding what facilitation means; it involves and the skills and personal attributes required by a practice developer to support change in day surgery units. Facilitation within the day surgery unit should focus on asking individuals or teams to analyse the area of innovation and change by:

- describing the identified issue/ activity
- identifying key collaborators, partners and team members
- discussing and agreeing on the vision, values and belief with the DSU context and culture
- negotiating tools and techniques for moving innovation and change forward
- consensual agreeing objectives and action plan
- negotiating time framework
- preparing and educating the team for implementation and evaluation

The above criteria are critical in order to repeat elements that are effective and to share knowledge with others and the future developments within the day surgery unit. To this end it is essential that individuals, teams and organisations familiarise themselves with ways of evaluating innovation and change in the day surgery unit.

Evaluation of innovation and change

A vital component in the cycle of practice development is determining its effectiveness through assessment of quality or 'evaluation'. Evaluation according to McSherry and Warr (2008) is a major facet of demonstrating excellence in health and social care. The reality of achieving this in day surgery practice is in finding innovative and creative ways of demonstrating the impact, outcome, efficiency and effectiveness of an innovation, change, new role or service improvement. These aspects of evaluation according to McCormack (2006) remain both challenging and difficult to do. McCormack (2006:123) further argues that 'the next era of advancements in practice development should focus on developing methodologies, testing out implementing strategies (methods) and adopting systematic approaches for evaluating processes and outcomes.'

The way forward to enabling the above issues surrounding the utilisation of evaluation methods, systems, processes and outcomes is to highlight what evaluation means along with some practical ways of engaging with the different methodologies.

Defining evaluation within the context of PD and day surgery

Evaluation is defined by Clarke (2001) as

> making a judgement about the worth or value of something. This can apply in the case of the informal subjective assessments that are part of every day life, such as when we assess the aesthetic value of a work of art. It also refers to the formal, systematic evaluations undertaken by professional evaluators or researchers.
>
> (Clarke, 2001:5)

Clarke's (2001) definition of evaluation is relevant to PD, in particular, within the day surgery unit setting. This is because the definition focuses on the subjective and objective aspects associated with measuring efficiency and effectives of a innovation and or change in practice/service. As suggested by the Health Service Executive South (2007:30), 'evaluation can differ in scale from a simple audit to a comprehensive evaluation of all aspects of a particular practice'. Sound evaluation is linked to measuring the aims and objectives of a given innovation and change. The aim of evaluating should be centred on providing objective feedback in relation to performance, outcomes and efficiency. These in turn can inform the decision-making process, in order to enhance quality with a day surgery unit.

Evaluation of PD activities within the day surgery unit setting according to Health Service Executive (2007), McCormack et al. (2006), McSherry and Warr (2006), and McSherry and Bassett (2002) could be affected by several conditions which promote or hinder engagement these are briefly outlined below.

Asking the evaluation questions

- Whether it works?
- Why it works?
- For whom it works?
- Under what circumstances it works?
- What has been learnt to make it work?

(Health Service Executive South 2007; McCormack et al. 2006)

Selections difficulties

- How to access the information?
- What is the best tool to use?
- How to implement the tool?
- The difficulty in choosing an indicator tool which meets the requirements of the service.

Practice constraints

- Lack of time needed to complete and interpret the apparatus.
- The difficulty of obtaining objectivity by the individuals using the measurement tools.
- The costs, which can be incurred by bringing in outside agencies to perform such reviews of practice.

Interpretation difficulties

- What to do with the data when available?
- The inability to implement the findings once the results are available.

McSherry and Bassett (2002)

To develop an effective evaluation framework within the day surgery unit, facilitators of change need to be able to identify and resolve the potential internal and external conditions (obstacles/barriers) that are associated with measuring and evaluating practice. The way forward for doing this is to ensure that you develop an evaluation strategy built into the project, change or service improvement/evaluation.

Prioritising and establishing a strategy for evaluation

McCormack et al. (2006:125) suggest that 'practice development evaluation frameworks need to embrace the methodological principles of participation, collaboration and inclusivity'. To ensure the development of an evaluation strategy that is both efficient and effective in capturing these important elements within your innovation and change it might be worth asking the following practical questions.

- What do I mean by evaluation?
- What do I want to evaluate?
- Why should an evaluation be done?
- What support/resources are there available to aid the evaluation?
- How will I share and disseminate the findings of the evaluation?

In response to the questions above, you may find that there are selection difficulties, practical constraints and/or organisational factors such as a lack of support/resources influencing what, how and why to evaluate the impact on patient outcome, services and or performance. As part of an evaluation it is important to decide on what you are evaluating. For example, do you focus on '*Impact assessment*'? – that is, determining the impact or changes that could be attributed or differentiated as a direct or indirect result of the innovation and change. Alternatively, do you focus on '*Performance assessment*' – that is, reviewing the effectiveness of the change or project in aiding the organisation achieve targets or standards laid down by government or detailed in given policies or standards like the National Service Frameworks. From our experience in PD, it is counter-productive to leave evaluation out of the designing/planning stages of a new innovation/change in practice. Evaluation is both a process and product, making it extricable to the furtherance of achieving quality services. The difficulties and challenges are how to prioritise and devise a strategy for evaluation.

Devising an efficient and effective strategy to evaluative practice (McSherry and Mudd 2005) should focus on identifying: the type of evaluation to be undertaken; structure; process or outcome, ensuring objectivity and consistency in the process and methods employed, differentiating the key components to be evaluated; clinical outcomes, service improvement, individual performance etc., and finally, evaluation should contain a staged approach: design, implementation, mid-term review, completion and sharing and dissemination. Some practical points to remember are:

- **Seek support:** you don't have to work in isolation link with the local university or research and development department!
- **Search and review the literature;** don't be afraid to build on the works of others!
- **Contact:** the people who have done it before locally, regionally and nationally and if necessary internationally.
- **Learn from experience:** talking and sharing with others who have contributed to the field.
- **Contribute:** be aware that you have something to share and disseminate, as part of your position, so networking and collaborating are essential.

Having identified the importance of developing a evaluation strategy, the next section highlights some evaluation methodologies that may support the process.

Evaluation methodologies

Evaluation of practice can be undertaken in variety of ways: clinical audit; patient satisfaction surveys; formal research, such as randomised control trials; non-randomised studies; descriptive studies; action research; review of guidelines and guideline development; utilisation of leadership and management style assessment tools and change models, to name but a few. To try and explain the relative merits and demerits of the various approaches and methods of measuring and evaluating practice would be unwise. What is worth pointing out at this stage is that the key thing is to access and apply the best approaches or methods to suit the innovation and change that you want to evaluate. For example, if an area of innovation and change involves a clinical team seeking the views of users for a given service, a patient satisfaction survey or research focus group could be used singularly or combined. Essentially, evaluation is about utilising the appropriate measurement or evaluative templates at the right time. Traditional approaches to the assessment of quality and developments have focused on the utilisation of audit tools, comparative benchmarking and patient satisfaction surveys.

Audit

The ultimate goal of audit according to Cooper and Benjamin (2004) is to improve patient care but additionally has the benefits of increasing professional knowledge, teamwork and communication, and of ensuring more effective use of staff time and resources. Audit contributes significantly to development of practice by offering a systematic approach to reviewing the outcome and quality of planned interventions. Johnston et al. (2000) reinforce the notion that despite many problems in its implementation, audit is now heavily rooted in professional practice within health and social care and is an essential element of Clinical Governance (McSherry and Pearce 2007). Lynn et al. (2007) argue that audit tools often measure the extent to which documentation has taken place rather than the implementation of developed skills and knowledge. Therefore within the day surgery unit it is imperative that audit reviews more than documentation but remain focused on patient outcomes. Indeed, Elliot (2006) suggests that the audit process is needed to determine whether clinical standards are being met, what those standards should be and how these will influence future practice and service developments.

Comparative benchmarking

Comparative benchmarking was introduced into the NHS as a requisite of *The New NHS: Modern, Dependable* (DH 1997) and instigated a rapid development of indicators and targets in health care, with the data collated from them being used for comparative performance assessment which could be compared across Trusts. Wait (2004) suggests that benchmarking is based on the premise that the public reporting of data will ultimately promote choice and the better use of resources resulting in improvement. Nutley and Smith (1998) indicated that the publication of indicators have several objectives:

- Secure accountability to funders and stakeholders
- Identify poor performance and excellence
- Help patients and purchasers chose providers
- Enable providers to focus on areas for improvement

An example of a day surgery unit bench marking tool is the Yardstick: Day Surgery Benchmarking Tool (2008).

The Yardstick Day Surgery Benchmarking Tool (Version 1.0) is a Microsoft Excel-based application, which allows users to compare Acute NHS Trusts' day case rates for the 25 day surgery procedures that make up the Audit Commission's 'Basket'.

Data for an individual Trust's Basket procedures can be displayed as a single bar chart, with each procedure's day-case rate compared against the national upper quartile rate, which is taken as a measure of reigning best practice. In the alternative case, for any given procedure, a Trust's day-case rate can be benchmarked against a user-defined peer group.

The graphical information that can be produced using the tool is intended to help key day surgery stakeholders, such as clinicians, managers and commissioners, to better understand what can be achievable as well as what the limitations to day surgery may be for a Trust with specific characteristics. More information can be found on the following web link:

http://www.dh.gov.uk/en/Healthcare/Secondarycare/Daysurgery/DH_4088193

To support day surgery units in moving forward with benchmarking, the Royal College of Nursing (RCN) (2007) offer some excellent guidelines for clinical practice benchmarking in order to develop practice. *A Model of Clinical Practice Benchmarking* (RCN 2007) is a benchmarking wheel containing twelve key points supporting practice to develop. These are as follows:

---

1.   Identity area of practice
2.   Expert input
3.   Patient focused outcome
4.   Identify measurement factor
5.   Identify benchmark of best practice and explore evidence
6.   Construct scoring method
7.   Score current practice
8.   Compare with best practice score
9.   Share examples
10.   Action plan
11.   Update
12.   Rescore

Adapted from RCN (2007)

By following the above framework, day surgery staff could easily apply this to support evaluation of existing practice. Benchmarking is useful way of highlighting and comparing performance within and between services and organisations for given standards/criteria of treatments and interventions.

Patient satisfaction

Richards and Coulter (2007) argue that to achieve one of the key goals of policy reforms and the Darzi (DH 2008) review making the NHS more patient-centred, patient experiences should be utilised in order to enhance care. National Patient Experience Surveys are now well established through the Healthcare Commission (HC) and are available to healthcare organisations (Coulter 2005). However Richards and Coulter (2007) believe that organisations should be conducting their own surveys in order to provide detailed feedback and focus on plans for quality and service improvements. Patient satisfaction should be demonstrated by reviewing patients' perceptions of implemented care. However, Larrabee and Bolden (2001) suggest that many implemented instruments are limited because they do not always consider the patients' experiences. Owens (1998) suggests that the incorporation of patient preferences when developing policies for clinical practice and patient assessment involving shared decision-making are integral aspects of patient choice.

The HC recommends that improvement of patient care and choices can be made by better use of feedback from patients. Lewis et al. (2000) argue that questioning patient satisfaction, comfort and system issues is a performance improvement initiative that has enormous nursing practice implications.

Wheeler and Grice (2000) argue that strategies used to generate patient (by extension user and, indeed, carer) feedback can include discovery interviews, focus groups, consultation meetings and questionnaires (both structured/unstructured), to name but a few. Questionnaires are the most common method utilised; strategically-placed suggestion boxes can generate good response rates and are of value in allowing service users to make suggestions and comments.

Conclusion

Practice development, though challenging and difficult, offers some fantastic opportunities in supporting innovation, change and evaluation within the day surgery unit contexts in the future. By embracing PD characteristics and qualities, and through utilising associated methods and methodologies, the quality and standards of care may be transformed within your day surgery unit. Practice development should not be optional but form part of everyone's role and responsibility, as part of their job description, contract of employment and professional code of practice in the quest for patient, public, person, people centeredness.

References

Audit Commission (2001) *Day Surgery: Review of National Findings – December 2001.* Audit Commission, London.

Arah, O.A, Klazinga, N.S., Delnoij, D.M., ten Asbroek, A.H. and Costers, T. (2003) Conceptual frameworks for health systems performance: A quest for effectiveness, quality and improvement. *International Journal of Quality Health Care*, 15 (5), 377–98.

Bassett, C. (1996) The sky's the limit. *Nursing Standard*, 10 (25), 16–19.

Bates, G. (2000) The challenge of practice development unit accreditation within an elective orthopaedic ward. *Journal of Orthopaedic Nursing*, 4, 170–74.

Clarke, A. (2001) Evaluation research in nursing and health care. *Nurse Researcher*, 8 (3), 4–14.

Clarke, C.L. and Wilcockson, J. (2001) Professional and organizational learning: Analysing the relationship with the development of practice. *Journal of Advanced Nursing* 34 (2), 264–72.

Collins, W. (1987) *Collins Universal English Dictionary*. Readers Union Ltd., Glasgow.

Cooper, J. and Benjamin, M. (2004) Clinical audit in practice. *Nursing Standard*, 18 (28), 47–54.

Coulter, A. (2005) *Trends in Patients' Experience of the NHS*. Picker Institute Europe, Oxford.

Department of Health (1997) *The New NHS: Modern, Dependable*. HMSO, London.

Department of Health (2002) *Day Surgery: Operational Guide: Waiting, Booking and Choice*. HMSO, London.

Department of Health (2007) *Our NHS our Future: NHS Next Stage Review Final Report Summary*. HMSO, London.

Dexter, F., Willemsen-Dunlap, A. and Lee, J. (2007) Operating room managerial decision-making on the day of surgery with and without computer recommendations as and status displays. *Anaesthesia and Analgesia*, 105 (2), 419–29.

Elliot, C. (2006) Clinical governance in gynaecological surgery. *Best Practice and Research Clinical Obstetrics and Gynaecology*, 20 (1), 189–204.

Foundation of Nursing Studies (FoNs) (2008) http://www.fons.org/dp/newsitems.asp (accessed 24 August 2008).

Garbett, R. and McCormack, B. (2001) The experience of practice development: An exploratory telephone interview study. *Journal of Clinical Nursing*, 10 (1), 94.

Glover, D. (1998) The art of practice development *Nursing Times*, 94 (36), 58–9.

Healthcare Commission (2005) *Acute Hospital Portfolio Review: Day Surgery*. Healthcare Commission, London.

Health Service Executive South (2006) *A Strategy For Practice Development*. Nursing and Midwifery Planning and Development Unit, Health Service Executive, Kilkenny, Ireland.

Hoban, V. (2007) Is practice development under threat? *Nursing Times*, 103 (24), 16–8.

Hynes, G. (2004) Exploring philosophical underpinnings for practice development education in Ireland. Paper presented at the 5th Annual International Research Conference, School of Nursing and Midwifery Studies, University of Dublin, Trinity College, Dublin.

Jackson, I. (2007) Day surgery overview: Where are we now, how did we get here and where are we going? *Current Anaesthesia and Critical Care*, 18 (4), 172–80.

JBI (2003) Management of the Day Surgery Patient, *Best Practice Supplement*, 1, 1–4.

Johnston, G., Crombie, I.K., Alder, E.M., Davies, H.T.O. and Millard, A. (2000) Reviewing audit: Barriers and facilitating factors for effective clinical audit. *BMA Quality in Health Care*, 9 (1), 23–36.

Kitson, A. (1994) *Clinical Nursing Practice Development and Research Activity in the Oxford Region*. Centre for Practice Development and Research, National Institute for Nursing, Oxford.

Larabee, J.H. and Bolden, L.V. (2001) Defining Patient-Perceived Quality of Nursing Care *Journal of Nursing Care Quality*, 16 (1), 34–60.

Lewis, C.K., Wahl, J., Yust, K. and Kaplan, S. (2000) *Journal of Perianaesthesia Nursing*, 15 (1), 12–9.

Lynn, M.R., McMillen, B.J. and Sidani, S. (2007) Including the provider in assessment of quality care: Development and testing of the Nurses' Assessment and Quality Scale – acute care version. *Journal of Nursing Care Quality*, 22 (4), 328–36.

McCormack, B. and Garbett, R. (2003) The characteristics, qualities and skills of practice developers. *Journal of Clinical Nursing*, 12 (3), 317–25.

McCormack, B. and Manley, K. (2003) Practice development: Purpose, methodology, facilitation and evaluation. *Nursing in Critical Care*, 8 (1), 22–9.

McCormack, B., Manley, K., Kitson, A., Titchen, A. and Harvey, G. (1999) Towards practice development: A vision in reality or reality without vision. *Journal of Nursing Management*, 7 (5), 255–64.

McPhail, G. (1997) Management of change: An essential skill for nursing in the 1990s. *Journal of Nursing Management*, 5, 199–205.

McSherry, R. and Bassett, C. (eds) (2002) *Practice Development in the Clinical Setting: A Guide to Implementation*. Nelson Thornes, Cheltenham.

McSherry, R. (2004) Practice development and health care governance: A recipe for modernisation. *Journal of Nursing Management*, 12, 137–46.

McSherry, R. and Driscoll, J. (2004) Practice development: Promoting quality improvement in orthopaedic care . . . as well as one's self. *Journal of Orthopaedic Nursing*, 8 (3), 171–8.

McSherry, R. and Johnson, S. (2005) *Demystifying the Nurse/Therapist Consultant A Foundation Text*. Nelson Thorne's Publishers, Cheltenham.

McSherry, R. and Mudd, D. (2005) Ways to evaluating the efficiency and effectiveness of the nurse/therapist consultant. In: *Demystifying the Nurse/Therapist: A Foundation Text*, (eds R. McSherry, S. Johnson) Nelson Thorne's Publishers, Cheltenham.

McSherry, R. and Warr, J. (2006) Practice development: Confirming the existence of a knowledge and evidence base. *Practice Development in Health Care*, 5 (2), 55–79.

McSherry, R. and Pearce, P. (2007) *Clinical Governance: A Guide to Implementation for Healthcare Professionals*, 2nd edn. Blackwell Publishing, London.

McSherry. R. and Warr, J. (2008) *An Introduction to Excellence in Practice Development in Health and Social Care*. Open University Press, McGraw Hill Education, Berkshire.

Manley, K., McCormack, B. and Wilson V. (2008) *International Practice Development in Nursing and Healthcare*. Blackwell, Oxford.

Meaden, S. and Solley, J. (2003) *Skill Mix and Nursing Establish For Day Surgery*. British Association of Day Surgery, London.

Mohr, J., Batalden, P. and Barach, P. (2004) Integrating patient safety into the clinical microsystem. *Quality Safety Health Care*, 13, 34–8.

Nutley, S. and Smith, P.C. (1998) League tables for performance improvement in Health care. *Journal of Health Service Research Policy*, 3 (1), 50–7.

O'Neal, H. and Manley, K. (2007) Action planning: Making your changes happen in clinical practice. *Nursing Standard*, 21 (35), 35–41.

Owens, D.K. (1998) Patient preferences and the development of clinical guidelines, *Spine*, 23 (9), 1073–9.

Page, S. and Hammer, S. (2002) Practice development: time to realize the potential. *Practice Development in Health Care*, 1 (1), 2–17.

Richards, N. and Coulter, A. (2007) Is the NHS becoming more patient centred? Trends from the national survey of NHS patients in England 2002–2007. Picker Institute Europe, Oxford.

Royal College of Nursing (2007) *Understanding Benchmarking: RCN Guidance for Nursing Staff Working with Children and Young People*. RCN, London.

Royal College of Surgeons of England (1992) *Guidelines for Day Surgery*. RSENG, London.

Wait, S. (2004) *Benchmarking: A Policy Analysis*. The Nuffield Trust, London.

Wheeler, N. and Grice, D. (2000) *Management in Health Care*. Stanley Thrones, Cheltenham.

Yardstick: Day Case Benchmarking Tool. http://www.dh.gov.uk./en/Healthcare/Secondarycare/Daysurgery/DH_4088193 (accessed 14 April 2008).

Day Surgery Management

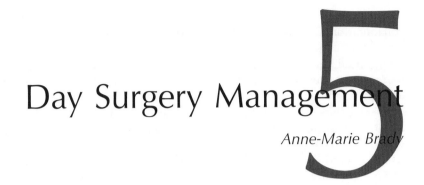

Anne-Marie Brady

Introduction

Day surgery includes all surgical treatments in which a patient is admitted and discharged on the same day (Healthcare Commission 2005). It represents a significant proportion of healthcare activity, as up to 80% of all elective surgery can be carried out in such environments (Jarrett 2001). Day surgery can potentially contribute to increased efficiency in surgical throughput, reduced waiting lists and optimal use of available bed capacity. Therefore its use must be strictly controlled to ensure it is appropriately utilised (DH 2002; Healthcare Commission 2005; Wales Audit Office 2006). Leading and managing day surgery units present unique challenges for healthcare providers. This is a labour-intensive service, reliant on effective collaboration between healthcare workers across the patient care experience. This chapter will discuss management and leadership behaviours that support day surgery practice. Operational issues, human resource management, performance management, and fiscal responsibilities that arise in managing the provision of services are discussed.

Management structure

Day surgery services should have an appointed clinical leader with a consultant anaesthetist or surgeon background with responsibility for strategy direction, clinical governance, clinical leadership and standard setting in collaboration with the Day Services Manager (DH 2002; Cutter 2005). The most suitable appointee for Day Services Manager is from a nursing background, as nursing functions are integral at all stages of the patient journey and they are uniquely able to integrate the clinical and logistical aspects of this work (Penn 1996; Healthcare Commission 2005). This is a senior nursing management position, and ideally will share the responsibility for strategic planning, clinical leadership, and standard-setting with the clinical director in addition to assuming responsibility for day-to-day operations (NLIAH 2004). Such services will also require the skills of an experienced healthcare administrator with expertise in the effective management of waiting lists, admissions and patient throughput (DH 2002). A users' committee should be established to enable all stakeholders in the day surgery process to share ideas in relation to the continuous quality improvement in the service (AAGBI 2005). This type of steering group would provide representation of patients, payers, referring primary care doctors in addition to management and clinical staff (BADs 2003a; AAGBI 2005).

Systems thinking

Day surgery is dependent on a number of administrative and clinical functions, delivered by a range of health care personnel. If any one part of the system does not function effectively or is changed, the nature of the overall service is changed. Systems thinking takes a long-range perspective and enables the analysis of structures that underpin complex organisations (Senge 2006). It is reliant on a shared vision among employees who see themselves as active participants in the system in which they work: 'Everyone sees the whole, specifically from the perspective of the user and looks at patterns of events, rather than working in isolation' (NHS Modernisation Agency 2005a:16).

The central concept of systems thinking is 'that our actions create our reality' (Senge 2006:220). Innovative ideas in health care can sometimes fail because they conflict with deeply ingrained ideas and therefore we are limited to using approaches and thinking that are familiar. Senge (2006) argues that ingrained ideas are our 'mental models' and these shape how we act because they affect what we are. At times these are below our level of awareness and, because they remain unexamined, they remain unchanged. Organisations and managers that promote skills in reflection are more aware of these preconceptions and how they influence their actions. *The key is to understand the chains of causality, the sequence and mutual interactions of the numerous individual cause and effect relationships that underlie the system of interest'* (Sherwood 2002:70).

Systems thinking enables staff to objectify the management issues that impact on their work. It assists employees in overcoming personality or traditional barriers to examine their work honesty so that staff may work in harmony with their colleagues. It enables the discussion of the structural issues that affect performance in the workplace. Managers will be able to communicate the systemic implications of various actions that contribute to organisational outcomes (Sherwood 2002). This requires open disclosure and analysis of all aspects of the day surgery system to create organisational knowledge. Effective systems are reliant on a constant flow of information about the nature of its own performance. This feedback places managers and staff in the strongest possible position to take decisions that will stand the test of time.

Management and leadership

The delivery of a seamless patient journey experience is dependent on work environments where both management and leadership functions are used effectively by all relevant stakeholders. Management has been described as using resources effectively to achieve organisational goals and this process has four steps: planning, organising, directing and controlling (Huber 2000). Leadership may be described as the process by which an individual uses influence to achieve organisational goals. It is an interactive process, dependent upon cooperation and collaboration between leaders and followers (Huber 2000).

Managers in progressive day surgery services will communicate a common vision to establish direction in addition in planning and budgeting effectively. '*A shared vision enables people within organisations to be committed and is vital for a learning organisation because it provides the focus and energy for learning*' (Senge 2006: 192). Considerable organisation is required to ensure a seamless service, with appropriate use of staff, delegation and effective communication to achieve desired organisational goals. Sustained energy is needed to lead and enable all staff to respond innovatively and with the flexibility to meet the unique needs of day surgery clients.

Personal mastery is a key trait of individuals in systems thinking organisations (Senge 2006). These are individuals who have emotional maturity and are constantly seeking a clearer understanding of their work reality. Reflective staff will challenge their own assumptions and will be capable of appraising their own contribution and that of others accurately. Emotional intelligence has similar characteristics, as highlighted by Goleman (1998). The key components of emotional intelligence found in effective managers:

Self-awareness: Realistic individuals who have understanding of their own values and aspirations as well as being able to judge accurately their own strengths and weaknesses. These individuals are self-confident, can honestly assess themselves and will be capable of assessing the organisations in which they work.

Self-regulation: This is the component of emotional intelligence that enables individuals to be reasonable in the workplace, with appropriate control over feelings and impulses. These individuals are open to change and have the potential to create environments of trust and fairness where productivity is not negatively impacted by politics and infighting.

Motivation: Driven not only be external incentives, such individuals are uniquely internally motivated and will display both innate optimism and organisational commitment.

Empathy: This is an essential component, which enables one to understand both the needs of the users of the service and also those of the providers. This is of particular importance in day surgery environments, where the service is dependent on understanding of the patient journey and teamwork in order to provide a patient-centred service.

Social Skill: Social skill enables individuals to find common ground and manage relationships of particular importance as day surgery is reliant on teams that are responsive to change and capable of continuously developing and expanding services.

Self-management skills are evidenced in the three first three components of emotional intelligence while empathy and social skill are concerned with how one manages relationship with others.

Teamwork

Systems' thinking reinforces the concept of collective work and day surgery is uniquely dependent on effective teamwork. Healthcare workplaces are placing increasing emphasis on the interdependence of professional and support staff and the importance of teamwork (Huber 2000). Effective leadership and facilitation by managers and leaders will assist in the development of cohesive and successful teams. Teams go through four stages of growth before they are sufficiently established, each requiring facilitation and intervention to varying degrees (Tuckman 1965).

Forming: In this introductory stage, team members begin to get know one another. Members may be easily distracted and difficulty may emerge in getting to know the problems requiring to be addressed. Minimal work can get done at this stage. The manager will make introductions, clarify tasks and deadlines and help define roles.

Storming: Personal agendas are very strong at this stage, as all team members attempt to negotiate how the team will function. Work can be affected by considerable levels of argument and disunity at this stage. The manager is required to promote dialogue and build trust and guide the team with a focus on the shared vision.

Norming: This stage is characterised by an acceptance of the team and rules. Members begin to work cohesively and find common focus. Relationships improve and members find renewed energy. Managers will engage in delegation and fostering independence within the team.

Performing: The normal process of struggle is overcome. Individual members develop insight into one another and the team can finally achieve productivity. Managers responsibility will include monitoring and evaluating performance in addition to seeking out new goals and opportunities to be pursued.

Team productivity is influenced by member attributes, work ethic and available resources as well as the nature and type of service to be delivered. 'A high performing team is a group of people whose mental models are naturally in harmony, especially as regards fundamental values' (Sherwood 2002:184). Team members will see the contribution of their individual work to the overall unit and organisation vision. Promoting team learning towards the achievement of organisational goals is a key responsibility of managers in day surgery. Team learning is *'the process of aligning and developing the capacity of a team to create the results its members truly desire. It builds on the discipline of developing shared vision. It also builds on personal mastery, for talented teams are made up of talented individuals'* (Senge 2006:218). In addition to developing members with the right knowledge, skills and attitudes, environments which enable honest communication, trust and collegiality among employees will contribute to successful teamwork.

Planning day surgery services

Mission statement

The mission statement clearly outlines the organisation philosophy, objectives, and goals and will communicates the priorities and values that underpin the service (Huber 2000). It should reflect the core purpose of day surgery, articulate outcomes and be consistent with strategic planning of the overall organisation. It should emphasise both the client population and the teamwork by staff needed to achieve organisational goals.

Operational policy

The management team in day surgery should develop and continually update operational policies and procedures in relation to all activities. These operational policy and procedures should be formulated after consultation with all staff groups and stakeholders in the day surgery process (Penn 1996; NLIAH 2004; AAGBI 2005; NHS Modernisation Agency 2007) and should include the following:

- Mission, philosophy and objectives
- Description of facility and service
  - Hours of opening and session times
- Management structure & organisational chart
- Staffing profile
  - Staffing levels
  - Job descriptions
- Financial arrangements and contracts
- Description of the patient journey
- Patient documentation
- Pre-admission policies
  - Booking systems
  - Admission procedures
  - Patient selection criteria
- Protocols for patient care
  - Reception
  - Pre-operative
  - Operative theatre
  - Recovery
  - Post-operative area
- Discharge protocols
  - Patient information
  - Transfer of patients unfit for discharge
- Procedures for utilisation of theatre time
  - Allocation procedure
  - Cancellation procedures
  - Reallocation of session procedure
  - Notification of leave policy
  - Start and finish time policy
  - Guidelines on case-mix/order of operating lists
- Health and Safety procedures
- Equipment maintenance and replacement schedules

Target activity

Day surgery management teams will need to be capable of planning strategically so that their units are best placed to meet the increasing expectation in relation to performance in this area. Internationally, it is estimated that currently 40–80% of all elective surgery is carried out as day surgery, although considerable variation in productivity between day surgery units has been demonstrated (Audit Commission 2001; DOH&C 2003; Day Surgery Council 2004; Healthcare Commission 2005). In the UK, the NHS has established targets for day surgery and this has influenced the approaches and the types of facilitates in which day surgery may be provided. The Audit Commission in the UK has established a 'basket of procedures' that is regularly provided in day surgery and can be used to developed target based activity levels of up to 75% (Audit Commission 2001). The British Association of Day Surgery has also developed a larger 'trolley' of procedures' that may be provided in day surgery and can be used to benchmark services against one another (NHS Modernisation Agency 2007). The ability to expand those surgical procedures that may be provided in day surgery will be dependent on local analysis that is responsive to National Health Service planning.

It is essential that the service is planned and delivered with patient requirements at the centre of service planning. There is an image of day surgery as minor surgery and that service is confined to delivery in regular hours only, on a 9–5, Monday–Friday basis. In some areas there may be tendency to plan and use day surgery around the preferences of individual consultants, which is not the most appropriate use of these services. Considerable expansion in this service is already under way which greater diversity in procedures and even more complex surgery being undertaken with this care delivery model. In some areas procedures will be scheduled throughout the 24-hour working day, thus permitting the efficient use of services and maximising use of bed capacity. This is referred to as a 23-hour/59-minute admission. The combined efforts of management working collaboratively with surgeons, anaesthetics and nurses will enable potential targets of 80% of all elective surgery, undertaken as day surgery to be met (Jarrett 2001).

Process mapping

One of the key aspects in successful day surgery is consideration of the systems issues that can affect the patient journey. Critical determinants of quality in the patient journey can be considered through the use of process maps to consider the aspects of services that may impinge on the timely and safe progression of the patient through day surgery. 'A process is a series of connected steps or actions to achieve an outcome', (NHS Modernisation Agency 2005b:11). Each day surgery service should prepare its own process map that reflects all the personnel and procedures that affect the patient journey in their area (Healthcare Commission 2005). Illustrating the patient journey in this manner assists all stakeholders in understanding the indirect activities in relation to planning and communication that are essential in effective delivery of day surgery services. Excellent service provision can be achieved if patient flow is used to design services (NHS Modernisation Agency 2007). Services should be developed that understand the patient journey and flow from pre-operative assessment to discharge (Figure 5.1).

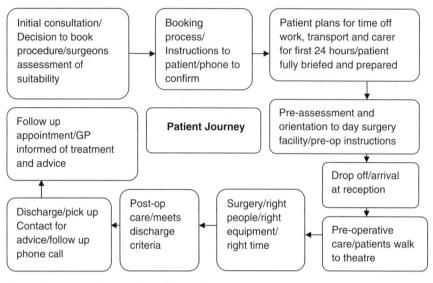

Figure 5.1   Sample Process Map of Patient Journey

Planning day surgery facilities

Health care is modernising and day surgery now accounts for an ever-increasing proportion of hospital admissions. The types of facilities that exist are influenced by the historical provision of care in addition to local resources, demographic profiles and geographical limitations. A variety of hospital-based and free-standing models exist for the provision of day surgery services in both the public and private sectors. Management need to evaluate the advantages and disadvantages of each type so they may be make provision for facilitating the patient journey as efficiently as possible.

Types of facilities

Independent dedicated day surgery facility with own operating room and patient-care areas with complete administrative responsibility for waiting lists and admissions.

Dedicated day surgery unit with dedicated operating room and patient-care areas within a larger organisation.

Day surgery unit with own patient-care areas within a larger organisation with use of main inpatient operating rooms.

Dedicated day surgery beds within main patient-care areas and use of main operating room. (Australian Day Surgery Council 2004; British Association of Day Surgery BADS 2003a; DH 2002)

The independent dedicated day surgery facility may be attached to a main hospital or be a free-standing building in either the private or public sector. It is the optimum day facility available and the advantage it offers is that patient throughput is not affected by competing demands in a larger organisation (DH 2002). The most cost-effective and ideal facilities for the provision of day services are a self-contained unit (NHS Modernisation Agency 2007), although the availability of such units differs in healthcare regions (Healthcare Commission 2005). This model enables providers to guarantee admission dates, and contributes to more effective planning, thus increasing convenience for patients.

In a dedicated day surgery unit within a larger hospital, there is exclusive use of an operating room, therefore patient flow is not affected by inpatient acuity issues. However, this type of facility is often reliant on the administrative support of the larger organisation which may result in less flexibility in response to cancellation or unforeseen changes in admission lists.

The day surgery unit is fit for purpose but is less than optimal, as it is influenced by competing demands of the main organisation. A large proportion of day surgery is still provided in departments which use the main operating room and admission procedures of larger organisations. This can negatively impact on efficiency as day surgery is competing with more acute needs throughout the operating day and will be classed as lower priority. When such services are required to use the main operating rooms of the larger organisation, the patient journey can be negatively impacted upon by systems issues that occur within the larger organisation. Indeed, use of inpatient operating room lists is not recommended unless the day case procedures are placed first on the list (DH 2002). Chapter 7 addresses admission procedures that provide positive experiences for patients and the organisation.

The use of inpatient beds for day surgery is the most inefficient approach and least desirable for managers in planning these services. As a result of competing priorities, inpatient needs will be favoured as these are more likely of greater acuity. Such systems are will be forced to prioritise acuity over efficiency. Therefore cancellations or delays causing unplanned additional admissions in such settings are not uncommon.

External facilities

Day surgery units require drop-off and pick-up points easily accessible to the unit in addition to easily accessible parking and wheelchair access (DH 2002). All facilities must be well signposted to guide patients to their destination with the least amount of distress possible. If day surgery services are to be utilised as the true 24-hour service envisaged, these facilities must be secure and well lit to facilitate out-of-hours access.

Internal facilities

The ideal facilities are purpose-built with emphasis on facilitating patient-centred throughput and maximum efficiency of services (NHS Modernisation Agency 2007). Administrative functions of day surgery are best delivered through dedicated personnel within such units, who have designated responsibly for contact, scheduling, throughput and follow-up with day surgery clients. This requires adequate space, technology, and appropriate and secure storage areas for medical records. A reception area with adequate waiting space for patient and relatives with ease of access and throughput is essential (NHS Modernisation Agency 2007). Also required, is the availability of pre-operative testing adjacent to the unit and adequate access to diagnostic equipment. This will provide opportunity for patients to familiarise themselves with their surroundings, reducing arrival delay and stress on day of surgery. The pre-operative and post-operative areas will be responsive to the needs of patients and may have a mix of equipment of beds and reclining chairs, depending on individual patient requirements. It is recommended that day surgery patients stay on one trolley during admission and that transfer of unconscious patients be avoided (DH 2002). There may be dedicated operating rooms which will require the provision of similar standard of equipment that may be anticipated in a main operating room. The availability of recovery beds must be at least one per operating room, but must also be able to respond appropriately to anticipate throughput. Day surgery services should also be situated as near as possible to pathology, pharmacy, X-ray and sterilising equipment and include adequate provision of staff rest and changing facilities.

Information management systems

Modernisation of information systems in health services are enabling opportunities for the creation of approaches to documentation that are integrated and common to all members of the multidisciplinary teams. There is increasing movement now towards the use of integrated care pathways by all members of the multidisciplinary team, which lend themselves to this type of centralised patients' record (BADs 2004). The information management system needs to be capable of interfacing with existing data collection mechanisms within the organisation: for example, X-ray, laboratory and ultimately GPs information management systems. There is need for access to computerised technology for all staff, in line with the development of a patient's electronic record (NHS 2006). This will minimise duplication and error within the system.

If the vision of day surgery as a 24-hour service is to be realised, day surgery information systems will require admission and booking procedures that can recognise the difference between a one-night inpatient stay and a planned elective admission, under the 23-hour/59-minute route (DH 2002). Information systems may be utilised to create templates of procedure times, to assist in optimum use of funded operating room time; basic timings can be identified by calculating the maximum time it takes an individual surgeon or anaesthetist to perform common procedures and a template can be generated in 80% of instances (NHS Modernisation Agency 2007).

Human resource management

Skill mix and staffing

The configuration of staffing in day surgery will be influenced by the nature of the patient referral and acceptance onto the day surgery service. Staffing levels will also be determined by the design of the facility, work undertaken and local preferences (AAGBI 2005). Other considerations in the allocation and recruitment of staff will include the types of case-mix and the expected throughput and capacity. The Healthcare Commission (2005) reported that those day surgery facilities that have their own operating theatre, have on average one whole time equivalent member of staff per staffed bed, trolley or reclining chair. There may be variable use of agency and bank staff depending on patient activity and local practice. Wide variation in productivity between day surgery units has been reported but productivity is increased per whole time equivalent in larger units (Audit Commission 2001).

The service may require dedicated consultant surgeons and anaesthetists, depending on the nature of the facility, with emerging career opportunities in the field known as surgical practitioner (Box 5.1). Nursing staff will be required at all stages of the patient journey, including pre-assessment, pre-operative, peri-operative and post-operative, and for follow-up triage, with use of operating room assistants and operating department practitioners

---

Box 5.1 Day surgery team

- Day surgery manager
- Clinical director
- Administrative, clerical and reception staff
- Registered nurses, ODAs and ODPs
- Medical staff – anaesthetist and surgeons
- Physiotherapist
- Health-care assistants
- Housekeeping staff
- Transport / portering staff.

Box 5.2   Staff allocation per shift *(BADS: 2003b:5)*

- In charge coordinator: experienced nurse per shift
- Pre-operative assessment: 1 nurse for 20 patients (approximately 20 minutes per patients
- Pre-and post-operative area; I nurse and IHCA per 7 patients
- Anaesthetic room: 1 nurse or ODA/ODP per session
- Operating room: 3 nurses/ODPs per session or per theatre (5 hours of nursing time per 4 hour list to allow for preparation and finishing)
- Recovery: 1 nurse per 2 patients (paediatrics 1 per patient)

---

depending on area of practice. Operating room practitioners (ODPs) in the United Kingdom pursue a two-year diploma professional registration course which equips them with skills to engage in the anaesthetic, surgical and recovery phases of patient care. Health Care Assistant (HCA) personnel provide supportive functions, which may include patient care, stock control, theatre assistance, and instrument maintenance (BADS 2003b). Day surgery services require dedicated housekeeping and transport staff to enable the efficient turnover of clients. Emerging models are multipurpose support workers who will provide elements of the former in addition to HCA activities. Box 5.2 outlines a typical staff for clinical personnel on one shift (BADs 2003b).

Evaluation of multiple factors will inform the determination of appropriate staffing ratios and skill in day surgery (NHS Modernisation Agency 2007; BADS 2003b), including:

- Exact nature of the patient journey
- Specialities, case mix and profile of patients
- Types of anaesthesia to be used
- Waiting list management
- Theatre utilisation information
  - Number of operating rooms
  - Allocated operating time
  - Start and end time of operating sessions
  - Anticipated volume of patients
  - Number of recovery spaces.

Selection and recruitment

It is critical for the day services nurse manager to be actively involved in the selection and recruitment of new members of the day surgery team. In selecting staff to work in day surgery, it is useful to consider key skills that are required by nurses or ODPs. These areas require staff with energy, motivation, and initiative, capable of adapting to a changing work environment. The work may be interpreted as predictable but requires staff to accurately organise and prioritise, and predict potential outcomes for clients. This is a fast-paced environment, where practitioners are routinely required to make effective clinical judgements and decisions in relation to patient discharge. Confidence in assessment is required to enable nurses to manage discharge needs appropriately. All individuals who work in day surgery need to be able to communicate effectively within a team environment with colleagues, patients and carers.

Multi-skilling

Day surgery lends itself to a client-centred models of care delivery. The ideal clinical staff will be multiskilled with capacity to rotate across all areas of day surgery service as appropriate (NHS 2003). Benefits of multiskilling include increased staff satisfaction, improved competency, increased cohesiveness and motivation within the team, as the staff are appropriately trained and understand each other's roles and responsibilities (BADS 2003b). Staff who are flexible and have experience of the entire spectrum of day surgery will be well placed to guide patients; an additional benefit is the increased coverage for sickness and absence that this staffing model affords. Rotation of staff is especially difficult in day surgery services where there is no dedicated operating room and patients interface with main operating rooms for that phase of service. This means that some staff may not be so readily transferable form one area to another.

Professional development

A primary function of management in day surgery services is to provide support and assistance to staff to enable them to maintain and develop their knowledge, skill, and competency so that they actively contribute to organisational development. Professional development should include competency-based education and training to enable staff to gain generic competencies in all areas of day surgery (DH 2002). Staff should be encouraged to participate in professional organisations such as the British Association of Day Surgery and the National Association of Theatre Nurses. Performance appraisal is both a formal and informal, interactive process that provides a forum by which organisational and individual goals may be discussed and aligned. This cyclical process includes the assessment of needs, setting objectives, agreeing the time frame for achievement and evaluating progress (Huber 2000). There are a number of post-registration courses that may be pursued by nurses to gain specialist knowledge that will inform practice in day surgery settings. These include peri-operative and day care nursing, theatre nursing, anaesthetics and peri-operative nursing.

Managing the provision of services

Managing waiting lists

Day surgery administration is more efficient when it is localised to the day surgery facility (DH 2002). Services are most efficiently utilised if the waiting lists are centrally managed within the day surgery services rather than by individual consultant or their secretaries (NLIAH 2004). A key management issue in day surgery is the implementation of good administrative practices to ensure services are appropriately utilised. Effective scheduling will enable treatment of the maximum number of patients which will reduce waiting times and maximise the potential of such facilities (NHS 2003). The provision of individual appointment times with adequate time to enable patients to make arrangements will limit cancellations and non attendance. Arrange ments and procedures to make contact with patients to remind of them appointments will also help reduce risk of non-attendance.

It is recommended that the lists of procedures that are performed in day surgery are reviewed frequently to ensure that services are being utilised appropriately (NHS 2003). Using such facilities for endoscopies and other non-surgical procedures may be an inefficient uses of resources. These procedures may be more appropriately facilitated in an outpatient environment, as they do not require sterile operating theatres or anaesthesia (NLIAH 2004; BADs 2003a).

Delegation

Care coordination is an important aspect of managing day surgery services. Delegation is the transfer of selected tasks and responsibility for completion of tasks to another person, and retaining supervision and accountability for that activity (Hansten and Jackson 2004). In all heathcare environments there has been considerable effort to redesign approaches to work, with the result that there are significant changes in the skill levels of those assigned to patient care. There is increasing attention to developing multiskilled workers and increasing use of unlicensed personnel in care delivery. These developments and indeed working in team-oriented environments with staff of different skills and abilities, requires considerable skill in delegation. Good delegation encourages innovation in subordinates, and most importantly frees the delegator to perform other tasks.

The *Five Rights in Delegation* can assist decision-making in relation to appropriate use of delegation (National Council of State Boards in Nursing 1995).

Right task: Is this task appropriate to delegate to another?

Right Circumstances: Appropriate patient setting with consideration of available resources and all other relevant information.

Right person: Is this right person delegating the task to the right person to be performed on the right person?

Right direction: Is the process of communication clear, concise, and does it clearly define objectives and anticipated outcomes?

Right supervision: Is there provision for monitoring, evaluation, intervention as required and feedback?

Time management

Effective managers evaluate constraints on time and foster work habits that use time productively (Grohar-Murray and DiCroce 2003). The Healthcare Commission (2005) reported that on average 24% of operating time in day surgery can be lost due to sessions not starting on time or finishing late. Managing planned operating-room time and creating time management practices that limit the unnecessary gaps between procedures in day surgery is essential to ensure an efficient and patient centred service. The next patient procedure should be ready to commence as soon as the previous patient has been escorted to the recovery room. Careful planning and utilisation of theatre time will minimise risk of delay in patient progress. For example, placing general anaesthetics before local will maximise time for patient recovery and reduce potential of insufficient recovery to enable patient to go home as planned.

Outcomes management

The importance of the active involvement of clinicians in all aspects of the service has been emphasised (Audit Commission 2001) with a common focus of shared values, goals, and objectives for all stakeholders. Healthcare policy has emphasised the devolution of authority for decision-making to include clinicians who are most familiar with services. Organisational knowledge is created in systems thinking workplaces (Senge 2006). Outcomes management involves a multidisciplinary approach to gathering information and making appropriate adjustments or changes in service provision. This enables the provision of quality care, control fragmentation, enhance outcomes and constrain costs (Huber 2000). It is not sufficient for health care providers merely to demonstrate that care was delivered:

consumers, employers, and payers demand evidence of appropriate utilisation of day surgery services reflective of national and regional service planning in relation to patient activity.

The patient journey in day surgery is complex and multifaceted. Key performance indicators should be collected and reported by all day surgery services (Healthcare Commission 2005; IAAS 2003). Successful outcomes management will depend on the production of appropriate data to enable managers and staff to reflect on and evaluate the performance of their units, determine priorities, and ensure value for money. Performance measurement is an important management tool to highlight areas where improvements in the service can be made. Transparency in documentation to attribute cause for the unplanned interruptions or delays in service will contribute to ongoing analysis and development of services. Valid and reliable measures related to performance are known as critical indicators (Huber 2000) and the following critical indicators that should be periodically evaluated in day surgery services (Audit Commission 2001; IAAS 2003; Healthcare Commission 2005; Wales Audit Office 2006; NHS Modernisation Agency 2007).

'Activity levels'

The number and nature of procedures provide baseline information for providers and payers in relation to the utilisation of services and will inform decision-making in relation to service planning (NHS 2003). There should be a clear distinction between true day cases and endoscopies or outpatient local anaesthetic procedures (BADs 2003a; Audit Commission 2001). There may also be national or local requirements for coding and documentation of activity. Demographic, clinical and administrative information from the medical record is coded in standardised format to facilitate analysis. Diagnostic-Relation Group (DRG) or Healthcare Resource Group (HRG) systems are used to classify hospital admission according to diagnosis and use of hospital resources (ESRI 2007; NHS 2003). The International Classification of Diseases is used for coding patients used in many countries (ESRI 2007). The Hospital-Inpatients Enquiry Scheme (HIPE) and the Hospital Episodes Statistics (HES) are national coded computerised databases of discharge summary information of acute hospitals (ESRI 2007: NHS 2007). The READ system used in United Kingdom combines International Statistical Classification of Disease and Health Related Problems (10th revision) and the Office of Population Census Surveys (OPCS) to code treatment and procedures in the NHS (NHS Modernisation Agency 2007). This provision of timely and accurate information on case-mix activity can be used to inform planning and service provision, quality improvement programmes and negotiating budgetary allocations.

'Did not attend rate'

This is the percentage of all day case patients who did not attend without giving notice (Healthcare Commission 2005). This is of critical importance: it represents a waste of resources as operating slots are vacant with insufficient opportunity to reallocate leading to an under-utilisation of services (Audit Commission 2001). The 'did not attend rate' can be further classified according to reason for non-attendance, including acute medical condition, patient decision or organisational reasons (IAAS 2003). This enables managers to understand systems issues such as problems with scheduling or approaches to patient information which may be causes of patients not presenting for surgery as planned. The recommended levels of DNA rate should be <2% and there should be a policy of reallocation of cancelled sessions (NHS 2003).

'Stay in rate'

This is the percentage of patients who require admission to inpatient beds rather than the anticipated discharge home (Healthcare Commission 2005). This has important resource implications as it means that inpatient beds are being inappropriately utilised. It is also a potential source of anxiety and dissatisfaction for service users who anticipate discharge home. A small percentage will be evitable due to unforeseen complications but well coordinated days surgery services should ensure this is kept to a minimum: less than 2% is recommended (NHS 2003). Further classification of 'stay in rate' for surgical reasons, anaesthetic/medical reasons or social/ administrative reasons is recommended by the IAAS (2003). Effective analysis of these types of occurrences can enable the day surgery team to examine and seek ways to improve scheduling, anaesthetic or surgical approaches which may be hindering the patient's ability to be discharged as anticipated.

'Cancellation on arrival'

This represents the percentage of patients where procedures are cancelled after arrival at the day surgery facility (DH 2002). This will include the documentation of reason for cancellation including pre-existing medical condition, acute medical or organisational reasons (IAAS 2003). Analysis of these types of events can highlight problems that may have occurred in relation to patient instructions or indeed inappropriate selection or assessment of client for day surgery.

Re-admission rates

This represents the percentage of patients who have an unplanned return or readmission to the day surgery facility or hospital (IAAS 2003). This can be further analysed by consideration of the time period following discharge

- <24 hours
- >24 hours and <28 days

Careful consideration of instructions to patients or indeed procedures for follow up by the day surgery management team can assist in reducing such occurrences.

Theatre utilisation information

Information on the use of operating-room time should be collected regularly as this will enable managers to evaluate efficiency within the service (Table 5.1).

Patient care indicators

Effective planning with attention to detail in relation to patient care will minimise the waiting times for patients, avoid cancellation, unnecessary

Table 5.1 Theatre Utilisation (*Adapted from: National Leadership and Innovation Agency (2004) Innovations in Care:* Good Practice Guide for Day Surgery, *NHS Wales*)

Operating room time	Note
Maximum available capacity	Maximum amount of operating time that would be possible if all session were fully funded, booked and utilised
Planned time	Amount of time planned to be used and represents the capacity that can be offered
Allocated time	Amount of funded operating available taken into account planned leave, maintenance, and reallocation of lists to other users
Available used time	The number of hours that took place. Audit Commission Acute Hospital Portfolio (2000) target: 92.5–95%
Agreed list start and actual start item	All staff should be aware of agreed time and variances between the two represent lost time
Agreed list end and actual end time	Agreed time last patient should have the left the operating room.

delays and maximise capacity. Patient satisfaction and clinical outcomes will be enhanced by good patient information systems. Appropriate follow-up arrangement will reduce potential for inappropriate usage of health services following discharge. The following indicators should be regularly audited to facilitate measurement of good practice in day surgery (Audit Commission 2001) (Box 5.3).

Box 5.3   Indicators of good practice in patient care *(Audit Commission,* Day Surgery *Appendix 2 2001:16)*

1. Are patients given a specific date and time for procedure when the decision to go ahead with the procedure is taken?
2. Are patient given individual appointment times or booked to arrive in blocks through out the day?
3. Are patients contacted in advance by telephone to remind them of their appointment?
4. Are patients seen and assessed for procedure between the decision to admit and the day of the procedures?
5. Are patients given written material in advance, before the day of their procedures?
6. Does the written material include
    a) what to expect when they arrive at the day surgery unit, with a description of the procedure and the sequence of events that will take place in the unit?
    b) who to contact for further help and advice?
    c) who to contact if they have a complaint?
7. Are patients given written information at discharge?
8. Does the written material at discharge include
    a) advice on what to expect that specifically addresses the procedure they have had and information on likely speed of recovery and common problems?
    b) advice on how to delay with common postoperative problems, such as control of pain, nausea and vomiting, with advice as to what to do for themselves and when to seek further advice?
    c) a telephone number at the hospital for queries and emergencies
9. On discharge, are patients telephoned when they are at home to check progress?
10. Have you conducted a patient satisfaction survey in the last two years (this is defined as a questionnaire or interview given to a minimum of ten patients asking them about their experiences whilst in the care of your unit)?

Financial management

Budget

A budget is a planning process that expresses in quantitative terms the revenues and expenses that may be anticipated for the coming year (Neumann and Boles 1998). It communicates the plan of activities and serves as mechanism for monitoring expenditure and measuring performance. A budget will express the anticipated workload, predict the required staffing and estimate the finance that will be needed pay for resources to achieve that workload (Bailey 1996). The process of financial planning and budgeting involves decision making in relation to the appropriate allocation of resources (Huber 2000). The management team is expected to ensure value for money, predict projected spending accurately and keep spending on staffing, equipment and supplies within budget. A completed budget has several component parts:

Revenue Budget: Demonstrates revenue and the sources of reimbursement based on statistical information derived from patient activity. Prospective payment systems operate in many day surgery facilitates where standard reimbursement rates are negotiated according the Diagnostic Related Groups (DRGs).

Operating Budget: Demonstrates anticipated spending for the coming year. Day surgery is labour intensive and staffing will account of the largest portion of anticipated spending. This budget will include supplies, service contracts and maintenance.

Capital expenditure budget: This is usually considered separate to the operating budget and demonstrates the spending that will required for the purchase of buildings or equipment that will be used for more than one year.

Costs: Revenue budgets in day surgery are often calculated with specific targets in relation to number of procedures and patient turnover. It is necessary to understand the costs or expenses than are incurred in generating revenue, so that costing of day surgery services is accurate. Managers are generally only held responsible for direct costs within their control.

Direct costs: are those that may be specifically traced to a particular procedure or service and can be attributed directly to a responsibility centre (Sullivan 2006). Salaries and surgical materials are categorised as direct costs.

Indirect costs are those that are apportioned across the organisation and can not be traced to a particular procedure or service (Neumann and Boles 1996). Management salaries and administration in day surgery are examples of indirect costs.

Variable costs are those costs that vary with volume or activity (Neumann and Boles 1996). Surgical supplies and use of agency or bank staff will vary in day surgery according to patient activity.

Fixed costs do not change with changes in volume or activity (Sullivan 2006). Many indirect costs such as management salaries or long term maintenance contracts are also fixed costs.

Responsibility cost centres

A responsibility cost centre is an organisational unit for which a manager has assigned responsibilities for activities (Neumann and Boles 1996). Depending on area of employment, day surgery managers may have varying degrees of supervisory responsibility and budgetary responsibility for the service they oversee. Managers will monitor and sign off on all spending attributed to their cost centre.

Monitoring the budget

Managers of specific cost centres are responsible for overseeing the budget operation and for variance analysis (Grohar et al. 2003). This process provides a mechanism for evaluating both department and managerial performance. A budget variance is the difference between the budget and actual expenditure. (Bailey 1996). Managers will be required to submit written explanation of both positive and negative variances. Ongoing variance analysis provides insight into planning for the next year.

Service/business plans

The preparation of an annual service plan is a means to integrate programme objectives and performance requirements and should utilise the principles of strategic management (O'Sullivan and Butler 2002). Planning for the future development of services or re-negotiation of existing reimbursement of services is a key management concern in day surgery. In negotiating contracts and reimbursements for services, the day surgery management team will be required to produce business plans or service plans at least annually or each time a service is renegotiated.

Conclusion

There is variation in the rates of day surgery performed and the approaches to the delivery of day surgery services (Healthcare Commission 2005; Wales Audit Office 2006). Systems thinking and teamwork is essential to the provision of day surgery services. The accurate measurement of performance outcomes by management will enable the ongoing development of existing and new capacity within day surgery services. Negotiation of contracts and marketing of day surgery services requires budgetary skill for management. Successful management of human services and ongoing provision of services will enable the provision of a quality day surgery experience to more patients, with improved access, reduced waiting times and increased consumer and staff satisfaction.

References

Association of Anaesthetists of Great Britain and Ireland (AAGBI) (2005) *Day Surgery*, revised edn. http://www.aagbi.org (accessed 24 August 2008).

Audit Commission (2001) *Acute Hospital Portfolio on Day Surgery: Review of National Findings.* http://www.audit-commission.gov.uk/ (accessed 24 August 2008).

Australian Day Surgery Council (2004) *Day Surgery in Australia: Report and Recommendations of the Australian Day Surgery Council*, revised edn. http://www.surgeons.org/Content/NavigationMenu/WhoWeAre/Affiliatedorganisations/AustraliaDaySurgeryCouncil/Day_Surgery_in_Austr.htm (accessed 2 September 2008).

Bailey, D. (1996) Budgeting skills. *Nursing Standard*, 10 (19), 43–8.

British Association of Day Surgery (BADs) (2003a) *Commissioning Day Surgery: A Guide for Primary Care Trusts.* http://www.daysurgeryuk.org/content/files/Handbooks/Commissioning.pdf (accessed 24 August 2008).

British Association of Day Surgery (BADs) (2003b) *Skill Mix and Nursing Establishment for Day Surgery.* http://www.daysurgeryuk.org/content/files/Handbooks/SkillMix.pdf (accessed 24 August 2008).

British Association of Day Surgery (BADs) (2004) *Integrated Care Pathways for Day Surgery Patients.* Colman Print, Norwich.

Cutter, T.W. (2005) The Role of the Medical Director. *Journal of Ambulatory Surgery*, 12 (1), 7–9.

Department of Health (2002) *Day Surgery Operational Guide: Waiting, Booking and Choice.* http://www.dh.gov.uk/PolicyAndGuidance/OrganisationPolicy/SecondaryCare/DaySurgery/fs/en (accessed 24 August 2008).

Department of Health & Children (2003) Press Release: *Waiting list data.* http://www.dohc.ie/press/releases/2003/20030522.html (accessed 3 September 2008).

Economic and Social Research Institute (2007) *Hospital Inpatient Enquiry Scheme (HIPE).* http://www.esri.ie/health_information/hipe/ (accessed 3 September 2008).

Goleman, D. (1998) What makes a Leader? *Harvard Business Review*, 76 (6), 93–102.

Grohar-Murray, M.E. and DiCroce, H. (2003) *Leadership and Management in Nursing*, 3rd edn. Prentice Hall, New Jersey.

Hansten, R. and Jackson, M. (2004) *Clinical Delegation Skills: A Handbook for Professional Practice*, 3rd edn. Aspen Publication, New York.

Healthcare Commission (2005) Commission for Healthcare Audit and Inspection. *Acute Hospital Portfolio Review.* http://www.healthcarecommission.org.uk/_db/_documents/04018392.pdf (accessed 24 August 2008).

Huber, D. (2000) *Leadership and Nursing Care Management.* W.B. Saunders Company, United States of America.

International Association for Ambulatory Surgery Management (2003) *International Association for Ambulatory Surgery: Universal Clinical Indicators for ambulatory surgery.* http://iaas-med.com/modules/content/index.php?id (accessed 24 August 2008).

Jarrett, P.E. (2001) Day Care Surgery, *European Journal of Anaesthesiology*, 18 (23), 32–5.

National Council of State Boards in Nursing (1995) *Delegation, concepts and decision-making process.* National Council Position Paper. http://www.nursys.com/public/resources/ncsbn_delegation.htm (accessed 24 August 2008).

National Health Service (2003) *Day Surgery Planning Toolkit.*

National Health Service Modernisation Agency (2005a) *Improvement Leaders Guide: Working in systems process and systems thinking.* www.institute.nhs.uk (accessed 3 September 2008).

National Health Service Modernisation Agency (2005b) *Improvement Leaders Guide: Process mapping, analysis and redesign – general improvement skills.* www.institute.nhs.uk (accessed 3 September 2008).

National Health Service (2006) *Guidance for NHS about accessing patient information in new and different what and what this means for patient confidentiality.* http://www.connectingforhealth.nhs.uk/systemsandservices/nhscrs/publications/staff/nhsguidance.pdf (accessed 3 September 2008).

National Health Service HES Online (2007) *Hospital Episodes Statistics.* http://www.hesonline.nhs.uk/Ease/servlet/ContentServer?siteID=1937&categoryID=537 (accessed 24 August 2008).

National Leadership and Innovation Agency for Healthcare (NLIAH) *Day Surgery: A Good Practice Guide.* http://www.wales.nhs.uk/sites3/docmetadata.cfm?orgid=484&id=40941 (accessed 3 September 2008).

National Leadership and Innovation Agency (NLIAH) (2004) *Innovations in Care: Good Practice Guide for Day Surgery.* This and the previous query are on the same site. http://www.wales.nhs.uk/sites3/docmetadata.cfm?orgid=484&id=40941 (accessed 3 September 2008).

Neumann, B.R. and Boles, K.E. (1998) *Management Accounting for Healthcare Organisations*, 5th edn. Precept Press, Illinois.

O'Sullivan T.J. and Butler, M. (2002) *Current Issues in Irish Health Management.* IPA, Dublin.

Penn, S. (1996) Day Surgery Management and Organisation. In: *Principles in Day Surgery Nursing,* (eds S. Penn, H.T. Davenport, S. Carrington, M. Edmondson), pp. 13–27. Blackwell Science, Oxford.

Senge, P.M. (2006) *The Fifth Discipline: The Art and Practice of the Learning Organisation.* Random House Business, London.

Sherwood, D. (2002) *Seeing the Forest for the Trees: A Manager's Guide to Applying Systems Thinking.* Nicholas Brealey, London.

Sullivan, D.W. (2006) Financial Outcomes. In: *Leadership Competencies for Clinical Managers* (eds A.M. Barker, D.T. Sullivan, M.J. Emery), pp. 251–71. Jones and Bartlett publishers, Massachusetts.

Tuckman, B.W. Development Sequence in Small Groups. *Psychological Bulletin*, 63, 384–99.

Wales Audit Office (2006) *Making Better Use of NHS Day Surgery in Wales.* www.wales.nhs.uk/documents/WAO_Day_Surgery_Eng_web.pdf (accessed 24 August 2008).

Communication Issues in Day Surgery

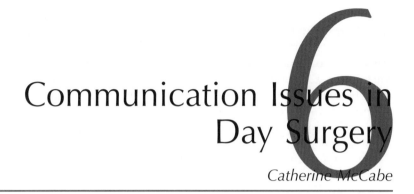

Catherine McCabe

Introduction

Day surgery has been an integral part of healthcare services for many years, and is regarded as an efficient and effective way of facilitating large numbers of patients receive treatment, quickly and with minimum disruption to their lives. With developments in technology and drugs, it continues to evolve as the hub of the delivery of surgical procedures in health care today. This chapter explores how communication plays a key role in providing a positive experience and high quality care for patients before, during and after day surgery. This will include discussion in relation to models of communication and how they relate to the day surgery context. The challenge of getting to know patients and delivering care in a therapeutic manner in the busy and transient environment associated with day surgery units is explored. The last part of this chapter looks at the importance of collaboration in providing patient-centred, efficient and safe day-care surgery and the communications skills needed to make it successful.

Communication

There is little doubt that communication is an integral part of the work of nurses and many authors agree that positive communication is the foundation stone in providing high quality nursing care in any clinical situation (Attree 2001; Thorsteinsson 2002; Wilkinson 1999). However, for many of us, communication is an unconscious process, therefore, we don't think about our communication behaviours and how they influence others. This does not generally cause problems but it may result in a lack of self-awareness and this influences how we contribute to patient care and service provision on a personal and professional level.

Many authors have attempted to define communication but this chapter is not so much concerned with defining it as with explaining its key components and discussing how knowledge of these provide understanding of why communication plays such an important part in the outcomes of nurses' interactions with patients and colleagues.

Communication theories may not have a direct influence on how people communicate but by exploring and discussing them, it is possible to identify patterns of communication behaviour. In a nursing context, communication theories can illustrate the differences between task-centred and person-centred communication. Linear models of communication, for example, depict communication as a one-way process involving a person sending a message and a person receiving the message (Berlo 1960; Miller and Nicholson 1976).

Message

Sender → →→→→→ Receiver

Although this model of communication is clear and contains two key elements of the communication process, it fails to acknowledge other influencing factors, the main one being the interpersonal interaction that occurs. Others include subjective or intrinsic factors such as individual values, beliefs, role, knowledge and goals; and extrinsic factors, such as the physical environment, organisational culture and semantics (McCabe and Timmins 2006).

Communication models that include the key components of the communication process, and also acknowledge the complexities involved, include the 'Circular Transactional Model of Communication' (Bateson 1979) and 'A Skill Model of Interpersonal Communication' (Hargie and Dickson 2004). Clearly Hargie and Dickson's (2004) skills model of interpersonal communication is more contemporary than Bateson's (1979) model, however, both models acknowledge the intrinsic and extrinsic factors listed above that influence the communication process and both models include the dynamic and evolving nature of communication in any given context. The key components of the Circular Transactional Model of Communication are:

- Intrinsic factors that influence the sender and receiver
- Extrinsic factors such as distracting stimuli and channels of communication
- Interpersonal space
- Context and environment.

Hargie and Dickson (2004) include the following factors in their Skills Model of Interpersonal Communication:

- Person-situation context
- Goal
- Mediating processes
- Response
- Feedback
- Perception.

This model includes and expands on many of the issues outlined in the Circular Transactional Model of Communication. It understands and incorporates issues that are particularly relevant to nursing, for example, it refers to issues of self-efficacy (belief in one's ability to succeed) and established boundaries. These are issues that nurses' need to understand and considering how to improve and develop communication skills. Traditional hierarchical systems exist in many areas of health care and nurses need to understand how these influence their communication behaviour and professional development in order to overcome them. Hargie and Dickson (2004) suggest that personal and professional self-awareness is essential in order to prevent negative communication and outcomes in interactions with others.

Exploring and discussing models of communication may seem a world away from reality and a busy day surgery unit but taking time out to consider such models will help nurses clarify the key components of the communication process and the complex and dynamic way in which these components interact and influence their day-to-day work. Some nursing models based on communication and interactions acknowledge these components and support both Bateson's (1979) and Hargie and Dickson's (2004) models. These models include Fosbinder (1994), Morse et al. (1992) and Morse et al. (1997) and they focus exclusively on the nurse–patient relationship.

Fosbinders's (1994) model is based on feedback from patients which indicated that patients considered the nurses' interpersonal abilities essential in having a positive experience. They identified information giving, getting to know them, establishing trust and going the extra mile as key components in a successful nurse–patient relationship. In the context of day surgery, this means assessing the individual needs of each patient before giving information and ensuring that they are ready and confident about going home after their surgery.

The model given by Morse et al. (1992) is based on emotional engagement. It suggests that a nurse can use either patient-focused or nurse-focused communication which is described as being either spontaneous or learned. It is a useful model because it illustrates the different communication behaviours that nurses use and may help in the development of self-awareness. Patient-focused behaviours that are spontaneous or learned include sympathy, compassion, humour, reassurance and comforting. These communication responses are patient-centred and when used by nurses, make patients feel cared for and treated like an individual (McCabe and Timmins 2006). Nurse-focused behaviours that are both spontaneous and learned include distancing, labelling, ritualistic practice, and false reassurance, for example, 'don't worry' and 'everything will be fine'. This type of communication is not patient-centred and can have a negative influence on the patients' experience of day surgery. When patients hear such phrases, it may make them feel that they are worrying excessively or over-reacting to their situation. This can result in patients becoming very anxious.

The Comforting Interaction Relationship Model (Morse et al. 1997) is presented in three parts. The first relates to how nurses act in terms of their styles of care and patterns of communicating based on their professional experience. The second part looks at patient actions in terms of how they communicate discomfort and distress to the nurse, recognising that patients also influence nurse–patient interactions by whether they decide to trust a nurse. The third aspect of this model relates to the evolving relationship between the nurse and the patient and suggests that the relationship needs to be negotiated as it develops, and is maintained and concluded.

It is clear from looking at these models that theoretically, that the relationship and context of the interaction are of equal importance as the individual contribution of the sender, message and receiver. Without considering and valuing the relationship and understanding the context, nurses cannot communicate in a patient-centred way. Exploration of these nursing and non-nursing communication theories may help nurses who are interested in developing and improving their communication to bring possible patterns of behaviour into their awareness.

Importance of communication in day surgery

Patient-centred communication is the foundation stone for providing effective and high quality care (McCabe and Timmins 2006; Cooper et al. 2002; Otte 1996), however, there are a number of factors to think about when considering communication issues in day surgery. These include the environment, the individuality of patients, the transient nature of their day surgery experience and the experience of day surgery itself. This starts at the assessment stage, pre-admission visits, surgery, and post-surgery recovery at home. As discussed in earlier chapters, each of these stages needs planning, organisation and expertise. As members of a multidisciplinary team, nurses are involved in each of these stages. In order to communicate effectively, they need to be aware of patient communication needs and how these change over the continuum of their day surgery experience. Like patients in any healthcare setting, information, education, and care that is individualised is valued by those in day care units. The challenge for nurses is how to provide this in such a transient environment where, on average, patients are physically present for a total of six hours but the information and support they receive from the day surgery unit before and after their surgery is as influential as their actual experience in the unit (Mitchell 2002). The complete day surgery experience for patients usually begins many weeks before the surgery and recovery can take anything up to two weeks. However, most research on patients levels of pain following day surgery do not record data beyond day three (Coll et al. 2004). Therefore, although nurses are involved at each stage, they may only see a 'snapshot' of the patients' experience, depending on where along the day surgery path they meet the patient. In order to develop communication skills that are therapeutic and patient-centred, nurses need to practice and over time it will become evident that, even in day surgery units where nurse–patient relationships are transient and of limited duration, time is not a factor in providing patient-centred and therapeutic communication (McCabe and Timmins 2006).

Therapeutic communication

The goal of therapeutic communication in nursing is to develop focused, purposeful, and positive relationships with patients in order to achieve mutually agreed outcomes of care (McCabe and Timmins 2006). Communication can only be therapeutic if patients feel secure and trust not only the nurses' professional skills and abilities but also perceive that the nurse has a genuine regard for them as individuals. McCabe and Timmins (2006) suggest that the key characteristics of therapeutic communication include active listening, openness, warmth, genuineness, empathy and professional skills. It is obvious that these communication behaviours are normal, everyday skills used by people either consciously or subconsciously. However, in a professional context such as nursing, these skills are used in a focused and purposeful manner. For nurses with a genuine regard for patients and concern for their individuality, being therapeutic is not difficult. Some nurses, however, may find this more challenging. This is not because they are not nice people or do not communicate as well, it is because they are focused on issues other than patients, for example, completing certain tasks. These tasks may be directly or indirectly related to patient care but what is absent is the patient-centred interaction. Nurses and other healthcare professionals can appear to be very busy people and although they may not mean to, the message they send (non-verbally) to patients is that they are too busy to talk. This non-verbal and task-centred approach to communication emerged as having a negative impact on the relationship between patients and healthcare professionals (McCabe 2004; Otte 1996).

The task-centred approach to nursing is not taught in undergraduate or postgraduate nursing programmes, despite the fact that, in clinical practice, the culture and socialisation of nurses has a direct influence on how care is delivered. As already mentioned, the day surgery environment, with its reliance on documented protocols, procedures and care pathways, delivery of care can be viewed as a matter of ensuring that all the boxes are ticked and protocols have been followed before a patient is discharged. This is an essential part of patient care and of ensuring patient safety; it is also a means of communication across the healthcare disciplines without direct interaction. The potential for falling into a task-centred approach greater with this system of care and the needs of the patient as a unique individual can be forgotten. It is clear that, in order to be therapeutic when communicating, the nurse must also be patient-centred.

The ability to be patient-centred depends on the organisational attitude and approach to planning, implementing and evaluating patient care services but perhaps more importantly and on a personal level, it is portrayed in the interactions between nurses and patients. According to Rogers (1961), qualities such as warmth, genuineness and empathy are a prerequisite for a nurse to be patient-centred. For nurses who are interested in developing patient-centred communication skills, self-awareness is essential. By becoming self-aware, a nurse can begin to bring personal beliefs, values and feelings into their general awareness and understand how their communication behaviours impact on colleagues and patients. This will allow them to recognise the value that they place on the relationship they have with patients and indeed with their colleagues and respond in a patient-centred way rather than based on their own needs and experiences. The process of becoming self-aware requires personal commitment, honesty and persistence. Introspection, seeking and reflecting on feedback from others are the key behaviours required in order to become self-aware (Siciliano 2005). Although generally regarded as a personal journey, individual self-awareness as a foundation stone has the potential to contribute enormously to professional and service development. The NHS Modernisation Agency Leadership Centre (2005) reports that leaders who are aware of how they communicate and are sensitive to how this impacts on others and influences work situations are more likely to be successful in collaborative endeavours.

Getting to know the patient

Getting to know the patient may be perceived differently depending on whether it is from the nurses' or patients' perspective. Nurses need to know the patients medical status, whether all correct procedures have been carried out before surgery and ensure that the patient is informed and ready for their surgery. This is done through a process of information giving and education that is provided verbally and non-verbally (information leaflets). However, according to Mitchell (2002), as the scope and availability of day surgery procedures, and developments in anaesthesia expands, the greater the onus is on the patient to self-care. This is accompanied by levels of direct contact with nursing and medical staff that are reduced when compared with being an inpatient. This has implications for the way in which nurses communicate with patients and whether patients perceive that nurses get to know them as individuals. As we have seen in other chapters in this book, day surgery units use documented policies, procedures and protocols to ensure efficiency and patient safety and this facilitates nursing and medical staff to deal effectively with the high patient turnover. It is important, therefore, to be aware that in an environment where standards, policies and documents such as integrated care pathways or core care plans are used to deliver care, it is likely that individual patient needs can be overlooked. If this happens, patients will feel anxious and vulnerable (McCabe 2004; Gilmartin 2004). In their framework for person-centred nursing, McCormack and McCance (2006) report that person-centred outcomes of care include satisfaction with care, involvement with care, feeling of wellbeing and creating a therapeutic culture. They suggest that these outcomes are achieved by working with the patient's beliefs and values, engaging with patients on a personal level, providing for patients' physical needs and sharing decision-making. The prerequisites for being successful in these actions are identified as being professionally competent, self-awareness, being committed to nursing and having developed interpersonal skills. It is clear that nurses need to get to know their patients so that they can interact with them and provide care in a patient-centred way. There are a number of behaviours that nurses can use to get to know their patients while also conveying a sense of genuine interest and concern for them. These include establishing rapport, questioning and collaborative communication.

Establish a rapport

Establishing rapport with patients is an essential communication skill in nursing because it allows the patient to decide if they trust the nurse. Having trust in the nursing staff will help to reduce patients' anxiety levels. Active listening is a key ingredient in developing trusting relationships and also allows a patient to see when a nurse has a genuine interest in them, both as an individual and as a patient who needs their care and attention (McKay et al. 1995). The first step a nurse must take if they wish to demonstrate active listening is to stop what they are doing and look at the patient. This may require only a moment or two and establishing eye contact, smiling and asking open and closed questions will allow a trusting and mutually satisfying interaction to take place. Active listening may require a nurse to give their complete attention to a patient but it does not usually require more time (McCabe 2004; Astedt-Kurki and Haggman-Laitila 1992; Williams 1998). Practising these skills will demonstrate this, as over time, the active listening behaviours become the normal and most frequently used communication behaviour. Gilmartin (2004) suggests that, given the transient and high-turnover context, healthcare professionals need to take responsibility for ensuring patient-centred communication is used in day surgery units. Foy and Timmins (2004) support this view and suggest that when a nurse demonstrates a concern for patients' knowledge, feelings and experience, it is perceived by patients as being patient-centred and therefore, therapeutic.

Questioning

Use questioning to establish the patients' level of knowledge regarding their forthcoming surgery. Some patients need and want more information than others and this should be considered planning and delivering their care (Kopp and Shafer 2000). Too much or too little information may only add to their already raised levels of anxiety and the process of getting to know the patient is essential in assessing and evaluating their individual needs. Using open and closed questions has a number of functions, it allows the nurse to gather information he/she needs, it gives the patient an opportunity to raise any concerns they have, and it is a medium through which the nurse can get to know the patient. This will only be successful if the nurse uses active listening skills, otherwise, the patient may not trust the nurse and therefore, will not be interested in developing a relationship. Asking a simple question like, 'Do you have any concerns about going home?' is an example of how to reassure patients and provide care that is patient-centred.

Some of the nursing care of patients who have undergone day surgery takes place over the telephone, when the nurse phones the patient at home the following day, or if the patient phones the day surgery unit with a concern regarding their recovery. Active listening is important in this situation also and although eye contact is not possible, the use of open and closed questions is still very effective. However, in these situations, the nurse needs to use a steady, moderate tone of voice and be careful not to sound busy or rushed, which may prevent patients from voicing their concerns and result in them feeling dissatisfied and anxious (Gilmartin 2004; Otte 1996).

Collaborative communication

So far in this chapter, the discussion has centred on nurse–patient interaction and relationships. However, in order for a patient to experience patient-centred care, there is another communication skill to consider and that is collaborative communication. It is clear from the other chapters in this book that in order to develop protocols, policies and procedures for day surgery units, collaboration between health professionals, management and administrative staff is essential. This can be difficult to achieve due to the traditional hierarchical roles that exist in health care. Nurses by the nature of their work spend more time with patients than any other healthcare professional and this includes a key role in co-ordinating and implementing the care prescribed by other professionals. In addition to this, nurses provide nursing care that is prescribed by nurses. This means that nurses need to take a central role in the development of day surgery services at all levels in the health care system and this requires skills in collaborative communication.

Shortridge et al. (1986: 130) suggest that in a healthcare context, 'collaborative practice emphasises joint responsibility in patient care management, with a bilateral process of decision making based on each practitioner's education and ability'. Although a comprehensive definition, it fails, like many other definitions to convey the dynamic and complex components of collaboration in health care (Siegler and Whitney 1994). This definition centres on collaborative practice and does not include reference to collaborative interaction. Collaborative practice does not require a great deal of interaction between health care professionals but it is implicit that those involved, for example, doctors and nurses trust each other in terms of making decisions and seeking advice when appropriate (Siegler and Whitney 1994). This is important on a day-to-day basis and works well when care is guided by jointly developed protocols and procedures as in day surgery services. However, problems may arise when collaboration is required for the development of services. All relevant personnel are generally included in discussions when services are being developed, therefore it is essential that nurses use this opportunity to act as patient advocate and ensure that services are patient-centred.

Different models of collaborative practice exist but a look at two illustrated by Siegler and Whitney (1994) may help clarify the differences in underlying concepts and meaning. The first (Figure 6.1) represents a un-idirectional and hierarchical approach with the doctor directing the practice.

Figure 6.2 represents an interdisciplinary and patient-centred model with all concerned working together but with the patient at the centre of all

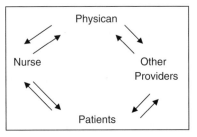

Figure 6.1　Unidirectional and hierarchical model of collaboration (*Reproduced with permission of Eugenia L. Siegler*)

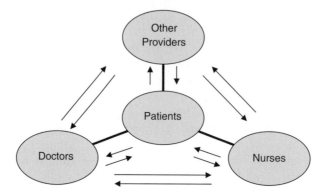

Figure 6.2 Interdisciplinary and patient-centred model (*Reproduced with permission of Eugenia L. Siegler*)

endeavours and no one health care personnel dominating the process. This is the ideal to which all collaborative practice and interaction should aim and is essential in the development of patient-centred practice and professional practice.

Before collaboration can be regarded as feasible or realistic, mutual respect, trust and tenacity on the part of those involved must be present (Kramer and Schmalenberg 2003). The next step in successful collaboration is to ensure awareness of the goals of the collaborative process by all involved. There are many reasons why collaboration is not successful in health care contexts. These include the socialisation of doctors and nurses as students and staff, poor communication, and power issues with the role of the nurse being perceived as 'invisible' in healthcare delivery by other health professionals and perhaps even nurses themselves (Lindeke and Sieckert 2005). A possible effect of this is that nurses find it difficult to contribute to decision-making processes in a confident and enthusiastic manner. However, collaborative communication is essential for collaborative practice, therefore, all nurses should aim for and actively work towards its achievement. The outcome of collaboration is improved patient care and a transformational day surgery practice (Kramer and Schmalenberg 2003; Siegler and Whitney 1994).

According to Malone and Morath (2001), emotional maturity is fundamental to allowing a person to engage successfully in collaboration because they are responsible, positive, focused and deal with difficult situations or failures in a constructive way. As mentioned in Chapter 5, self-awareness is an important tool for helping a person attain and maintain emotional maturity. It will also help nurses as individuals to realise that they have a personal responsibility to value collaborative communication and develop the necessary skills. Self-awareness means that individuals know and understand themselves and are aware of how their feelings, actions, values, attitudes and beliefs influence relationships and interactions with others. A person cannot begin to understand others until they are self-aware. Developing self-awareness is a lifelong process that requires introspection, critical reflection and acknowledging and actively seeking feedback from others. As a profession that is perceived by other healthcare professions and indeed by nurses themselves as inferior, it is essential that nurses begin to take responsibility individually and collectively for the development of the profession and its contribution to the development of healthcare services. This is particularly relevant to the day surgery context because of the dramatic expansion of available surgical procedures over the last decade. In order to ensure that day surgery services are patient-centred and meet the needs of individuals, nurses must be an integral part of the development and instigation of new and effective services. According to Easson-Bruno (2003), nurses need to demonstrate emotional maturity through their leadership and stop blaming others for problems or difficulties that exist in nursing. This prevents nurses from taking responsibility and being constructive in their approach to professional and practice development.

Assertiveness is another essential skill for effective collaborative communication. It also requires mutual respect in order to be successful. Balzer-Riley (2000) suggests that assertiveness is the ability to express thoughts, feelings and ideas with undue anxiety or having a negative effect on others. Characteristics associated with effective assertive behaviour are confidence, responsibility, consistency and the ability to use active listening skills effectively. It is well documented that nurses tend to demonstrate more submissive communication behaviours than assertive (McCabe and Timmins 2006), but this does not mean that they do not have the necessary skills, with the right amount of encouragement and support, we can all be frank, flexible and open-minded (Lindeke and Sieckert 2005). Assertiveness can be simple or confrontational and requires the use of specific communication behaviours, including to:

- demonstrate respect (active listening)
- be responsible, use 'I' statements
- make clear statements rather than questions
- use firm, moderate, consistent pitch/tone
- verbal/non-verbal communication need to match
- focus on present problem and address one point at a time
- offer feasible suggestions/solutions.

Simple and confrontational assertiveness are based on the same communication behaviours but are used in different situations and for different reasons. Simple assertiveness is used on ordinary, everyday interactions when a person merely states their opinion or needs. Confrontational assertiveness is more focused, in that it addresses specific issues directly and is essential in dealing effectively with conflict which often occurs in collaborative processes. Development of these skills and genuinely valuing and embracing collaborative communication also changes the way in which conflict is perceived. Freedom to disagree is essential in collaborative communication and is perhaps essential in order for it to be effective in bringing about lasting changes and developments in services. Although communication skills such as development of self-awareness and assertiveness are taught in undergraduate and postgraduate nursing programmes, nursing students can only value and use these skills if they see them used in the clinical areas. Role models using these communication skills to collaborate effectively in day-to-day situations and at a managerial and leadership level demonstrate the power and valuable role that nursing, along with other healthcare professions, have in providing patient-centred care. As we all know, it frequently takes just one person to obstruct proceedings and if this is allowed to happen often enough, then their effect can be permanent. Therefore, the presence of mature, focused leaders from all relevant professions with a common goal is essential to the success of all collaborative endeavours. According to Lindeke and Sieckert (2005) in order for collaboration to be successful, those involved need to establish common goals. Often doctors and nurses fail to collaborate effectively because they are motivated by different goals. However, by establishing a patient-centred focus as demonstrated in Model II (Figure 6.2), there is common ground to work from, with issues of hierarchy, economics, and politics coming second to sharing knowledge, skills and resources by all team members. It is important to acknowledge that although this chapter addresses day surgery from a nursing perspective, it is not assumed or expected that other healthcare professions possess the necessary attributes, values or beliefs necessary in order to participate in collaborative communication. Nurses need to be mindful of this when attempting to enter or establish collaborative processes.

Conclusion

Providing patient-centred care in any context requires patient-centred and collaborative communication. Due to the rapid turnover and transience of patients, this is particularly challenging in day surgery units. Understanding the various communication models, both nursing and non-nursing, will help nurses to begin to understand and identify their own communication behaviours. It is through this self-awareness that nurses can begin to develop not just the communication skills necessary for patient-centred and therapeutic care, but also for a collaborative communication with other health care colleagues. This is essential also for the provision and ongoing development of day surgery services that are patient-centred and cost-effective.

References

Astedt-Kurki, P. and Haggman-Laitila, A. (1992) Good nursing practice as perceived by clients: A starting point for the development of professional nursing. *Journal of Advanced Nursing*, 17 (10), 1195–9.

Attree, M. (2001) Patients' and relatives' experiences and perspectives of 'Good' and 'Not so Good' quality care. *Journal of Advanced Nursing*, 33, 456–66.

Balzer Riley, J. (2000) *Communication in Nursing*, 4th edn. Mosby, St. Louis.

Bateson, G. (1979) *Mind and Nature*, Dutton, New York.

Berlo, D. (1960) *The Process of Communication: An Introduction to the Theory and Practice*. Holt, Rinehart & Winston, New York.

Coll, A.M., Ameen, J.R.M. and Moseley, L. (2004) Reported pain after day surgery: A critical literature review. *Journal of Advanced Nursing*, 46 (1), 53–65.

Cooper, D.W., Garcia, E., Mowbray, P. and Millar, M.S. (2002) Patient-controlled epidural fentanyl following spinal fentanyl at caesarean section. *Anaesthesia*, 57, 266–83.

Easson-Bruno, S. (2003) Don't blame Florence [electronic version]. *Nursing Leadership*, 16 (4), 8–9.

Fosbinder, D. (1994) Patient perceptions of nursing care: An emerging theory of interpersonal competence. *Journal of Advanced Nursing*, 20, 1085–93.

Gilmartin, J. (2004) Day surgery: patients' perceptions of a nurse-led preadmission clinic. *Journal of Clinical Nursing*, 13, 243–50.

Hargie, O. and Dickson, D. (2004) *Skilled Interpersonal Communication: Research, Theory and Practice*. Routlege, Sussex.

Kopp, V.J. and Shafer, A. (2000) Anesthesiologists and perioperative communication. *Anaesthesiology*, 93, 548–55.

Kramer, M. and Schmalenberg, C. (2003) Securing 'good' nurse physician relationship. *Nursing Management*, 34 (7), 34–8.

Lindeke, L., Sieckert, A. Nurse-Physician Workplace Collaboration. Online Journal of Issues in Nursing, Vol. 10, No. 1, Manuscript 4. www.nursingworld.org/ojin/topic26/tpc26_4.htm (accessed 24 August 2008).

McCabe, C. (2004) Nurse–patient communication: An exploration of patients' experiences. *Journal of Clinical Nursing*, 13, 41–9.

McCabe, C. and Timmins, F. (2006) *Communication Skills for Nursing Practice*. Palgrave Macmillan, London.

McCormack, B. and McCance T. (2006) Development of a framework for person-centred nursing. *Journal of Advanced Nursing*, 56 (5), 472–9.

McKay, M., Davis, M. and Fanning, P. (1995) Expressing. In: *Bridges Not Walls*, (ed J. Stewart), 7th edn. McGraw-Hill, Boston.

Malone, G. and Morath, J. (2001) Pro-patient partnerships. *Nursing Management*, 32 (7), 46–7.

Miller, G. and Nicholson, H. (1976) *Communication Inquiry: A Perspective on a Process*. Addison-Wesley, London.

Mitchell, M. (2002) Guidance for the psychological care of day-case surgery patients. *Nursing Standard*, 16 (40), 41–4.

Morse, J.M., De Luca Havens, G.A. and Wilson, S. (1997) The comforting interaction: Developing a model of nurse-patient relationship. *Scholarly Inquiry for Nursing Practice*, 11 (4), 321–43.

Morse, J.M., Bottorff, J., Anderson, G., O'Brien, B. and Solberg, S. (1992) Beyond empathy: Expanding expressions of caring. *Journal of Advanced Nursing*, 17, 809–21.

National Health Service Modernisation Agency Leadership Centre www.executive. modern.nhs.uk/framework/personalqualities/selfawareness.aspx (accessed 24 August 2008).

Otte, D.I. (1996) Patients' perspectives and experiences of day case surgery. *Journal of Advanced Nursing*, 23, 1228–37.

Rogan Foy, C. and Timmins F. (2004) Improving communication in day surgery settings. *Nursing Standard*, 19 (7), 37–42.

Rogers, C.R. (1961) *On Becoming a Person*. Houghton Mifflin, Boston.

Shortridge, L.M., McLain, B.R. and Gilliss, C.L. (1986) Graduate education for family primary care. In: *Nurses, Nurse Practitioners: The Evolution of Primary Care*, (eds M.D. Mezey, and D.O. McGivern). Little, Brown, Boston.

Siciliano, E. (2005) *Emotions in the Workplace: Part Two: Principles for Leaders Dallas ASTD* (American Society for Training and Development). http://www. dallasastd.org/news/ASTD/Articles/emotion2.htm (accessed 24 August 2008).

Siegler, E.L. and Whitney, F.W. (1994) *Nurse-Physician Collaboration: Care of Adults and the Elderly*. Springer Publishing Company, New York.

Thorsteinsson, L.S.C.H. (2002) The quality of nursing care as perceived by individuals with chronic illnesses: The magical touch of nursing. *Journal of Clinical Nursing*, 11, 32–44.

Wilkinson, S. (1999) Communication: It makes a difference. *Cancer Nursing*, 22, 17–20.

Williams, A.M. (1998) The delivery of quality nursing care: A grounded theory study of the nurse's perspective. *Journal of Advanced Nursing*, 27, 808–16.

Providing Information and Support

Margaret McCann

Introduction

As outlined in previous chapters, day surgery involves the admission and discharge of patients on the same day. Patients are discharged with no overnight stay and are expected to manage their recovery at home with the assistance of family members or carer(s). Consequently, they are required to care for themselves both pre-operatively and post-operatively in their own home environment. In addition, day surgery services are provided within an environment of health care cost containment where there is a strong emphasis on providing a more efficient and effective service. In order to ensure the effective operation of a day surgery service, it is essential, therefore, that patients and carers receive pre-operative and post-operative education, information and support. Failure to do so could result in non-attendance, incorrect preparation for surgery, delayed recovery, overnight admission and an increased demand on primary health care services.

This chapter aims to increase understanding of the important role patient education has in the effective operation of a day surgery service. We will discuss the benefits education and information giving has on the management of pre-operative and post-operative anxiety and explore the principles and process of patient education. In addition, different methods of delivering education will be examined, including the development of written information material.

Day surgery and patient education

The last 20 years have witnessed an ever increasing demand for day surgery services, which account for 50–80% of all surgeries performed across developed countries (Pearson et al. 2004). Indeed, the NHS Plan (Department of Health 2000) predicted that 75% of all elective surgical procedures in England would be carried out as day cases. The Audit Commissions 1990 'basket' of day surgery procedures included 20 procedures. However, as day surgery becomes more popular this 'basket' of possible procedures has also expanded (Table 7.1). The British Association of Day Surgery has also recommended a number of procedures suitable for day surgery (Box 7.1). Consequently, there is a large variety of procedures available and for education and information giving to be effective there is a necessity to ensure that appropriate and relevant information is provided to patients.

You have only to look at your own healthcare area to observe that the complexity and variety of day surgical procedures continues to grow. Meeting local needs and advancements in minimal invasive surgery, laser techniques, anaesthetics and pharmacological agents have contributed to the ever-changing profile of the patient attending the day surgery unit. Furthermore, increasing numbers of patients previously deemed not suitable for day surgery are now eligible for and offered this service. All of which has implications for the provision of education and information to day service users and their carers.

Benefits of patient education

Patients undergoing surgery experience a number of anxieties, including fear of surgery, anaesthetic, pain, and of the unknown, as well as worries about their family. Over the last 50 years the area of patient education has been well researched, with seminal works providing a body of evidence that clearly illustrates the benefits of patient education on pre- and post-operative outcomes. Early researchers such as Hayward (1975), Boore (1978), Wilson-Barnett (1978), Wilson-Barnett and Osbourne (1983), Devine and Cook (1986) and Howard et al. (1987) noted that patient education reduced pre- and post-operative stress, anxiety and pain and increased self-care and independence on the part of the patient – all of which contributes positively to patient recovery. However, much of this research was focused on inpatients who were admitted for a number of nights and whose needs differ somewhat from day surgery patients.

Day surgery patients have similar anxieties to inpatients but also have additional fears, such as anxiety about post-operative care following discharge, which can be linked to the lack of contact with nursing staff and the provision of inadequate discharge information (Otte 1996; Mitchell

Table 7.1   Basket 2000 day surgery procedures (Audit Commission 2001)

1. Orchidopexy	Correction of undescended testes	**General**
2. Circumcision	Cutting away of foreskin of the prepuce	**surgery and**
3. Inguinal hernia repair	Repair of the outpouching of the abdominal sack	**Urology**
4. Excision of breast lump	Removal in whole or part of a lump in the breast	
5. Anal fissure dilatation or excision	Correction of a tear of the skin around the anus	
6. Haemorrhoidectomy	Removal of thickened tissue and veins inside the lining of the anus	
7. Laparoscopic cholecystectomy	Removal of the gallbladder by means of an instrument introduced through a small hole in the stomach wall	
8. Varicose vein stripping or ligation	Removal of crooked and incompetent veins in the leg	
9. Transurethral resection of bladder tumour	Removal of a tumour by an instrument inserted into the urethra	
10. Excision of Dupuytren's contracture	Removal of fibrous tissue under the skin of the palm that causes the fingers to become bent	
11. Carpal tunnel decompression	Incision in the wrist to relieve pressure on the median nerve as it passes into the hand	**Orthopaedics**
12. Excision of ganglion	Removal of a lump usually around the wrist, hand or foot	
13. Arthroscopy	The use of a thin fibre-optic instrument to look inside a joint for diagnosis and/or treatment	
14. Bunion operations	Straightening of the big toe and removal of bony overgrowth causing it to bend	
15. Removal of metal ware	Removal of pins or plates used to stabilise a fracture	
16. Extraction of cataract with/without implant	Removal of a cloudy eye lens and replacement with a synthetic one	**Opthalmology**
17. Correction of squint	Repositioning the muscle of the eyeball	
18. Myringotomy	Relief of glue ear by making a small hole in the ear drum to release pressure and inserting a tube to avoid recurrence	**Ear, nose and throat**
19. Tonsillectomy	Removal of the tonsils	
20. Sub mucous resection	Relief of nasal blockage caused by a bent cartilage in the middle of the nose	
21. Reduction of nasal fracture	Repositioning of the bone of the nose	
22. Operation for bat ears	Removal of skin and cartilage at the back of the ears	
23. Dilation and curettage/Hysteroscopy	Removal of tissue from the uterus	**Gynaecology**
24. Laparoscopy	Use of fibre-optic instrument introduced through abdomen for diagnosis/ treatment of internal organs, usually by gynaecologists	
25. Termination of pregnancy	Evacuation of the contents of the womb	

Box 7.1 **Procedures suitable for day surgery** *(British Association of Day Surgery, DH 2002)*

1. **Laparoscopic hernia repair**
Repair of abdominal hernias using minimally invasive keyhole technology
2. **Thoracoscopic sympathectomy**
Keyhole chest surgery to reduce excess sweating of the hands
3. **Submandibular gland excision**
Removal of the salivary gland under the jaw when affected by stones or inflammation
4. **Partial thyroidectomy**
Removal of diseased thyroid gland in the front of the neck
5. **Superficial parotidectomy**
Removal of the salivary gland in the cheek – usually for non-cancerous tumours
6. **Wide excision of breast lump with axillary clearance**
Breast cancer operation removing up to 1/4 of the breast, and the glands in the armpit
7. **Urethrotomy**
Division of narrowing/stricture in the outflow from the bladder, often through a telescope
8. **Bladder neck incision**
Division of the muscle in the bladder neck to relieve some cases of enlargement of the prostate gland
9. **Laser prostatectomy**
Shrinkage of some cases of prostate enlargement using laser
10. **Trans cervical resection of endometrium (TCRE)**
Removal of the lining of the womb through a telescope; to avoid hysterectomy in some cases of heavy periods
11. **Eyelid surgery**
Correction of drooping or deformed eyelids
12. **Arthroscopic menisectomy**
Removal of damaged knee cartilage using keyhole technology
13. **Arthroscopic shoulder decompression**
Use of keyhole surgery to correct abnormalities limiting movement at the shoulder joint
14. **Subcutaneous mastectomy**
Removal of swollen breast tissue in men, or some cases of very early cancerous changes in women
15. **Rhinoplasty**
Plastic reconstruction of deformity of the nose
16. **Dentoalveolar surgery**
Removal of impacted or complex wisdom teeth
17. **Tympanoplasty**
Repair of perforated ear drum

1997; Costa 2001). Day patients' experience of surgery involves a rapid turnaround, which includes being admitted, having surgery and being discharged on the same day. Within a very short period, patients and carers are expected to take control of post-operative care and recovery from healthcare professionals. Lack of education and information in this patient group increases their anxiety and impacts negatively on their ability to cope and plan for their discharge. For example, patients undergoing laparoscopic abdominal surgery who do not receive sufficient education and information in the management of post-operative pain may seek assistance post-discharge from primary health care providers or the day surgery ward, so increasing the workload in these service areas. Increased readmissions to hospital and a prolonged recovery period for patients may also occur. Patient education, therefore, benefits patients' experience of day surgery and ensures its efficient delivery (Otte 1996; Twersky et al. 1997; McHugh and Thoms 2002; Cox and O'Connell 2003; Watt-Watson et al. 2004).

The evidence suggests that pre-admission contact with patients and carers reduces patient anxiety and improves patient outcomes. The provision of specific and relevant information and education plays an important role in the achievement of these outcomes. This ensures that carers have the necessary knowledge to assist them during their hospital stay and recovery at home, for example, the provision of verbal and written information on an abdominal laparoscopic procedure. Providing education and information is not a one-off event, it is an ongoing process that needs to continue throughout the patient's stay, with particular emphasis at the time of discharge (Mitchell 2000a; Rhodes et al. 2006).

Challenges associated with patient education

As anxieties differ between inpatients and day surgery patients, so too does the nature of their stay in hospital. The reality of day surgery means that a patient's stay will be short, involving minimal contact with healthcare professionals, including the day surgery nurse. As there is increased pressure on clinical space within the day surgery unit, nursing staff are under increased pressure to admit and discharge patients in time-efficient manner. As a result, they have limited time to spend with patients. Consequently, there is insufficient time to get to know patients and provide detailed education. This is in contrast to inpatients, who have the time and opportunity pre- and post-surgery and prior to discharge to ask questions, have their concerns and queries addressed and gain additional information.

The education needs of day surgery patients are similar to inpatients; however they require additional education and information to enable them, within their own home environment, to manage their pre-operative preparation and post-operative recovery. Patient education will, therefore, enhance the self-caring abilities of patients and carers prior to and following the surgical procedure. Other challenges facing patients is their first point of contact with day surgery nursing staff. This varies between healthcare settings. In some instances, patients will meet the nurse for the first time on their admission to the day surgery wards. In other settings, the first point of contact is made at a pre-admission clinic.

All of these scenarios present the challenge of knowing what information is pertinent to patients and carers and providing this information within a given short time frame. In order to overcome these challenges, every opportunity and point of contact with patients needs to be used for education. In addition, innovative and creative means of providing patient education are needed in order to provide patients and carers with a working knowledge of how to self manage and plan their recovery at home. These include the use of:

- pre-admission clinics
- pre-admission visits to the day surgery unit
- pre-admission telephone screening
- the provision of written material prior to admission.

As day surgery patients are dependent on education and information in managing their own recovery, another challenge confronting them is receiving insufficient information to assist them in this process. The NHS, as far back as 1993, identified that lack of information was a problem area within day surgery. Dissatisfaction with information received leads to patients feeling unprepared for the day surgery experience, resulting in overall dissatisfaction with day surgery services. Lack of education and information continues to be an issue in the first decade of the 21st century, with recent research indicating that patients feel inadequately informed about the procedure and the day surgery experience in its entirety. Patients did not know what to expect pre-operatively, post-operatively and throughout their recovery period at home (Costa 2001; Richardson-Tench et al. 2005). Indeed, Mitchell (2000a), in a review of empirical studies examining the opinions of day surgery patients, notes that improvement of information provision was recommended in 57.6% of 99 studies reviewed.

Lack of education and information also has implications for carers. They may not be able to anticipate a patient's need for physical or psycho-social support in relation to possible outcomes associated with the surgical procedure. These outcomes include pain and its management during recovery and the impact the procedure has on the patient's ability to carry out activities of daily living. Carers who have insufficient information may not be able to assist patients, for example, in the management of shoulder pain following an abdominal laparoscopic surgical procedure. Taking time to provide education and information are seen as the prerequisites for enabling patients and carers to actively participate in the management of their own care (Majasaari et al. 2005). The Association of Anaesthetics of Great Britain and Ireland (2005) went so far as to recommend that day surgery patients be supplied at the pre-admission clinic with pre- and post-operative instructions supported by written materials.

The success or failure of day surgery service rests on the self-caring abilities of patients and carers. The challenge confronting the day surgery nurse is therefore to ensure that patients and carers receive sufficient detailed education and information to manage their care. Patients and carers need to fit day surgery into their busy lives, which requires forward planning and making necessary adjustments to their home and work environment. Patients and carers who do not understanding the important role they have in the day surgery process will be reluctant to engage or actively participate in their own care, resulting in poor outcomes for day surgery. The day surgery nurse needs to assess, as soon as possible, for any deficits in patients' self-care abilities. Once identified, these deficits can be rectified through the provision of information and education. Again, this requires the imparting of specific information to patients and carers, so empowering them to make informed decisions about their care during the recovery process (Young et al. 2000).

Multidisciplinary approach to patient education

Various medical personnel utilise the services of day surgery, resulting in different surgeons carrying out similar surgical procedures. Difficulties arise when views and opinions on the content and provision of patient information differ from surgeon to surgeon. Consequently, during a period of minimal contact with patients and carers, healthcare professionals including the day surgery nurse are placed in the unenviable position of trying to remember and reinforce patient information, which differs from consultant to consultant. This can lead to the provision of education and information that is conflicting and confusing. As a result, there is a need for a multidisciplinary approach to the provision of education and the development of written material.

In order to maintain patients trust and the credibility of healthcare professionals, information giving needs to be consistent across all members of the multidisciplinary team. All key stakeholders have an important role to play in the development of consistent information both verbal and written. This will require close collaboration between team members. The formulating of verbal and written information needs to be planned and structured. Time needs to be set aside so as to ensure that comprehensive discussions take place and agreement reached between team members. The key stakeholders in this process may vary between healthcare settings but normally includes representatives from the surgical consultant team, anaesthetist, day surgery nurse, physiotherapist, dietician, pharmacist, community healthcare nurse and a representative from patients' groups.

As part of the multidisciplinary team, nurses face many challenges in the area of day surgery. These include trying to establish a relationship with patients who have an eclectic patient profile and with whom they have minimal contact. It is widely acknowledged in the literature that day surgery nurses play a significant role in the provision of patient education and information. This role is also recognised by healthcare providers, surgeons and anaesthetists who accept that the experienced day surgery nurse can organise and deliver effective patient education and information especially during the pre-admission clinic (DH 2002).

Day surgery nurses need to be multiskilled and experienced, with good communication skills, enabling them to educate patients and carers effectively (DH 2002). As there is a rapid throughput of patients, nurses need to be motivated to get involved with them and ensure that they deliver correct education and information to patients prior to discharge. As contact time is minimal, nurses also need to use every opportunity to reinforce education and information already delivered. Nurses who are trained and educated in day surgery will have a sense of what the day surgical experience means for patients. An important component of that education involves an understanding and knowledge of teaching and learning and the various strategies that can be used in educating patients and carers. In this current healthcare climate, understanding and incorporating health promotion into care delivery is also an important role of day surgery nurses.

Day surgery nurses have to deal with a large number of patients who may be admitted for similar procedures. There is a risk, therefore, that the provision of information and education may be determined by the need to appease the masses and be based on what day surgery nurses perceive patients and carers need to know. This approach to education may become ritualistic and habitual where the same approach is used for all patients. Patients become dissatisfied when education and information is generic and not individualised. In order to avoid this occurring, there is a need to develop a more patient-centred approach whereby the provision of verbal and written information and education is more specific to the needs of patients. Using a framework such as integrated care pathways is one approach to providing an individualist approach to care. As outlined in previous chapters, integrated care pathways, while highly organised, need a degree of flexibility in order to meet the individualised needs of patients and carers. The framework must also meet the demands of a day surgery service that is constantly changing, fast moving and ever-expanding.

Integrated care pathways offer day surgery nurses the opportunity to demonstrate the contributions they make to the delivery of care and education to patients. The use of integrated care pathways address a number of the concerns raised by Butler et al. (2006), who suggest that not documenting the type of services nurses provide and the contribution they make to patient outcomes may compromise nursing and fail to demonstrate the deep connections nurses have with patients. Integrated Pathways offer the day surgery nurse the opportunity to record what education they provide, thus, making visible their role in patient education.

Patient education and management of anxiety

As outlined in the communication chapter, information giving and education are important components in the delivery of patient-centred care and are key to a successful nurse–patient relationship. It is also evident that information giving and education are central to patient-centred communication and the reduction of patient anxiety. Furthermore, patient anxiety is influenced by the degree of education and information patients receive prior to and during their admission to the day surgery unit.

Mitchell (2002) supports this view and indicates that the key component to the effective management of anxiety is the provision of a desired level of information and education be it simple, standard or extended. Information and education can be classified as being either procedural, behaviour or sensory and can also be linked to problem-focused coping or emotional-focused coping information.

Types of information giving to day surgery patients

Problem focusing coping information is the most common form of pre-operative information provided in the day surgery setting. It incorporates procedure, behaviour and sensory information. Day surgery patients are self-caring, consequently, encountering a number of challenges during the pre-operative and post-operative period. The provision of problem focused coping information will help patients and carers to make informed decisions and solve problems, so enhancing their self-care abilities (Mitchell 2005).

Cognitive strategies, relaxation and modelling are all examples of emotional focusing coping information. These are used when the stressor or cause of anxiety can not be changed, however, they enable patients to view the stressor in a more positive light (Watt-Watson et al. 2004). Cognitive strategies involve the use of mental strategies which help patients overcome anxieties they may have, for example, the possible negative outcomes associated with anaesthetics and surgery. In contrast, relaxation strategies include the provision of information on different techniques such as music therapy, relaxations methods, distraction and guided imagery. Richardson et al. (2005), in a systematic review on patient education in day surgery, concluded that distraction via music or short stories and relaxation techniques were shown to reduce patient pre-operative anxiety across a range of anxiety indicators. Finally, modelling incorporates imitating the required or desired behaviour, using such techniques as demonstrations, teaching sessions, reading hospital leaflets, viewing video presentation or viewing other patients. The provision of emotional focused coping information in day surgery, while not as evident as problem focused information is an area that day surgery units may consider developing in the future (Mitchell 2005).

Procedure information, also known as situational information (Box 7.2), needs to be procedure specific in order to address the individual needs of patients. This contributes to a patient-centred approach to education. Indeed, patients attending day surgery expressed a higher preference for procedure information (Bernier et al. 2003). As anxious patients only retain

---

Box 7.2   *Examples of procedure, behaviour and sensory information*

Procedural information:

- Pre-admission preparation
- Admission process
- Order of events once admitted
- Pre-medication
- Transfer to and from theatre
- Anaesthetic and induction process
- Medical equipment and technology used during admission
- Surgical procedure
- Pre- and post-operative nursing care
- Expected outcome from surgical procedure
- Recovery at home
- Follow up care and contact

Behaviour information:

- Stop smoking prior to surgery
- Reduce weight prior to surgery
- Adapting a certain position for the procedure
- Elevation of limb post-procedure
- Specific post-op exercises (upper/lower limb, pelvic)
- How to cough and breath effectively

Sensory information

- Sensations felt when anaesthetic drugs first enter the body
- May feel cold when first entering the operating theatre
- May hear loud noises when first entering the operating theatre
- After the anaesthetic, might hear things before being able to open eyes or move around
- May experience headache after surgery
- May feel light headed the first time standing up after surgery
- May feel certain type of pain post-procedure, such as shoulder pain post abdominal laparoscopic surgery

50–60% of information, it is essential that verbal procedural information is supported through the provision of procedure specific written material be it in the form of information leaflets or information sheets (Grieve 2002).

Behaviour information focuses on the behaviour or actions patients are required to undertake before, during and after the procedure (Grieve 2002). This form of information is crucial to the process of patients and carers becoming active partners in the delivery of day surgery care. Behaviour information (Box 7.2), also referred to as 'patient role information', is described by Bernier et al. (2003) as the second most sought-after information from day surgery patients.

Sensory information relates to information that informs patients of the possible sensations they might feel, see or hear during their time in the day surgery unit (Box 7.2). Bernier et al. (2003) indicated that this was the least preferred type of information. However, in this prospective study only 50% of patients recalled receiving this type of information from day surgery nurses. This could have possibly influenced their perceptions on the importance of this type of information. Sensory information also results in patients experiencing less fear and anxiety prior to, during and post a procedure (Grieve 2002).

Patients' preference for procedure, behaviour or sensory information needs to be ascertained during the assessment process. This assessment should also take into account the level of anxiety patients are experiencing. In addition, the degree of information to be provided needs also to be assessed as patients with a preference for minimal information can become anxious if too much information is delivered.

Levels of Information Giving

Patients differ in the level or degree of information they wish to receive. Some patients would like an extended level of information provided to them while others are quite happy to receive a basic level. Providing too much or too little information can increase the anxiety these patients groups are already experiencing. It is argued that patients preference for different levels of information reflects their coping style. There are two coping styles – vigilant or avoidant coping (Mitchell 2005).

Vigilant copers need to know everything about the procedure and the day surgery experience so requiring an extended level of information in order to manage their anxiety effectively. Too little information will elevate their anxiety levels. Mitchell (2000a) reports that vigilant copers who received only simple information were more anxious than those who received extended information. In contrast, avoidant copers would like just enough information to help them through the procedure. They require a minimal level of information and too much information will cause a marked increase in their level of anxiety. Mitchell (2000a) concluded that day surgery patients with either vigilant or avoidant coping, when paired with the appropriate level of information will experience less anxiety.

Both of these coping styles are described as being at the opposite ends of a continuum, so necessitating the nurse to assess where the patient sits on this continuum. Based on this assessment, the nurse can then determine what level of information the patient needs. It is important to note that coping styles should be continuously assessed as they can change over time (Mitchell 2000; Mitchell 2005).

Successful planning and implementation of education and information requires nurses to determine the patient's preference for problem focusing coping information or emotional focusing coping information; procedure, behaviour or sensational information and determine if the patient is a vigilant or avoidant coper. This assessment will determine the type and level of information given to the patient during their pre admission visit. Consequently, there is a need to have experienced nursing personnel with excellent communication skills to undertake the pre assessment interview. Using these skills the nurse can develop a therapeutic relationship with patients, which will enable them to get to know patients and determine their educational and information needs.

Furthermore, the need to provide different types and levels of information has implications for the development of written material. A summary of key information points needs to be provided in the first section of any written information. This will ensure that the avoidant copers obtains a basic level of information without having to read the complete leaflet, thus, avoiding increased levels of anxiety. Vigilant copers can acquire extended information by reading all of the written material so ensuring they have the necessary education and information to manage their anxiety.

Patient education process

Ultimately, the goal of patient education is to give day surgery patients a sense of control over the management of their recovery. Patient education achieves this by developing patients' and carers' confidence and competence in their ability to self-manage their care in both the pre- and post-operative phase of their journey through day surgery. Consequently, empowering patients and carers to become autonomous decision-makers who accept responsibility for the manner in which they use this education (Redman 2004, Bastable 2006).

Patient education is not a passive process of simply providing information. Patients cannot be coerced to learn; therefore, there is a need for patient education to be an active process. It involves the active interaction between patients, carers and day surgery nurses, all of whom are seen as equal participants in the education process. This process involves the amalgamation of two components, patient teaching by the nurse and learning by the patient. Bastable (2006) describes the education process as a framework for a participatory, shared approach to teaching and learning.

Patient education, learning and teaching

There is no universally accepted definition for patient education and information. Indeed, patient education has been used synonymously throughout the literature with patient teaching and patient information. Over the last 30 years, definitions of patient education have moved from a passive to a more active process which is linked to health related outcomes. Current definitions suggest that patient education is a process of assisting people to incorporate health-related behaviours (knowledge, skills and attitudes) into everyday life with the goal of achieving optimum health (Bastable 2006). For day surgery patients and carers this involves the acquisition of new knowledge and skills to enable them to become self-caring.

Learning is described by Bastable (2006) as a relatively permanent change in thinking, emotional functioning and behaviour. It involves patients learning new knowledge, skills or changing their attitudes and behaviours. For day surgery patients learning can occur at any time and during any interaction with professional healthcare staff. Learning can cover such issues as self-care activities, pre- and post-operative management, preparations for interventions that patients may experience in day surgery and issue relating to health promotion (Falvo 2004).

The primary goal of teaching is active learning by patients. It involves the transferring of information from teacher to learner with the hope that the learner will assimilate and utilise this information. Teaching is not a single act but a deliberative and intentional series of acts in response to an identified learning need. It can be planned and systematically arranged or informal and unplanned whereby every interaction with the patient is used as a teaching opportunity. For teaching to be effective the learner must be motivated and ready to learn within an environment that is conducive to learning. There is also a need to consider the literacy level, educational background, culture and language skills of the learner (Falvo 2004; Bastable 2006). In day surgery this requires the patient to be mentally alert, physically stable and not denying the need for the surgical procedure. In addition, development of written information material on day surgery needs to take into consideration the literacy levels of the patient population. Teaching activities need to be patient- and carer-focused. At the end of this process it is essential that teachers ascertain patients and carers understanding of what has been taught. The process of teaching and learning is integrated into all stages of the patients journey in day surgery.

Education process and the patient's journey in day surgery

A patient's journey through day surgery may vary between healthcare settings. Some patients may be directed to a pre-admission clinic straight from the outpatients' department. Others may receive an appointment to visit this clinic a number of weeks prior to their admission. Although not ideal, there continues to be a percentage of patients whose first encounter with the day surgery unit is on the morning of their admission. Whichever journey the patient is forced to take, it has implications for the manner in which they are educated and informed about their procedure.

Ideally, patients should start their journey at the pre-admission clinic (Mitchell 2000a; Audit Commission 2001; Healthcare Commission 2005). It is at this visit that the education process should commence. During this visit patients are assessed physically, psychologically and socially for their suitability for day surgery and their ability to self-care at home. Skilled nurses assess patients' preference for problem or emotional focused coping information and determine if patients are vigilant or avoidant copers. Based on this information, nurses can then decide on the level of education and information each patient needs to receive. The outcomes of this is a less anxious and well prepared patient (Mottram 2001). This is also the ideal opportunity not only to assess what patients already know about the procedure and the day surgery experience but also to identify their individualised learning and health information needs.

During the pre-admission assessment, nurses have the opportunity to provide procedure, behaviour and sensory information in order to meet the identified learning needs of patients. Box 7.3 outlines the educational areas that need to be explored with patients and carers during the pre-admission visit. It is also the ideal time to discuss with patients possible emotional focusing coping information, such as relaxation and distraction techniques. During the pre-admission assessments visits, patients and carers will also get the opportunity to visualise the day surgery facility and familiarise themselves with the hospital setting, environment and staff. This will reduce patients' pre-admission stress and anxiety. It is imperative that patients are admitted within three months of their visit to the clinic. If they are waiting longer than this, then a follow-up telephone call will have to be made to reinforce information that they had received.

Providing information and education for the first time to patients on the day of their admission is not idyllic. Patients will be very anxious about their admission and may have difficulty remembering the information giving to them during this stressful period. Indeed, providing new information to patients after a general anaesthetic (GA) is not a suitable time for the provision of information as the anaesthetic impairs patients' concentration, judgement and ability to recall information (Aspen Reference Group 1997; Dewar et al. 2003), all of which reinforces the importance of patients being

Box 7.3   Preadmission education

Details on day surgery facility

- Opening hours
- Telephone numbers
- Parking arrangements
- Advised what to bring with them
  - Dressing gown, slippers, medications currently taking, books, magazines, small change for telephone
- Advise on what not to bring
  - Leave valuables at home
  - Avoid wearing make-up, including nail varnish, on the day of admission
- What time to arrive
- What time surgery will take
- Estimate length of time in the hospital and timetable of events
- Estimate time to organise transport to and from hospital
- The importance of an escort and when to ask them to come
- Responsible adult assistance overnight and for up to 48 hours or longer, dependent on surgery
- Can not use public transport home

Details on pre-admission preparation

- Fasting times should be specified
- Rational for fasting should also be provided
- Preparation for anaesthetic
- Medications what to take and what not take prior to admission
- What to do if patient has cold or is ill

What to expect on the day of surgery

- Admission process
- Sequencing of events that will take place during the day

Details on proposed surgery

- Use of pre-operative surgery specific medication, for example sedation, eye drops for ophthalmic patients
- Transfer to theatre
- Brief description of the operating room and its equipment
- Anaesthetic – what to expect from anaesthetic
- What is the surgical procedure

What to expect during time in recovery

- Need for taking blood pressure, pulse, temperature
- Need for oxygen masks
- Need to inform patients that as part of preoperative education that pain control is easier to achieve if commenced early, rather than waiting until pain becomes unbearable – aim of this education is to assist patients in reporting pain promptly
- What to expect immediately after the surgery (as appropriate to specific procedure)
  - Wound size and site
  - Type of suturing material most likely used
  - bandages, slings, crutches
- Expected outcome of surgical procedure

What to expect at discharge

- Relevant verbal and written material will be given to the patient and carer (information booklet or leaflet that is procedure specific and addresses patient's need for information that is patient centred and relevant to their needs)
- Follow up appointment will be arranged
- Need for responsible adult to pick them up and for overnight care at home – 1st 24 hours
- Type of dressings to be used on wound, supply will be given
- Removal of sutures – when, where, who

What to expect on return home

- Outline recovery time needed. It is important that this is not understated as patients will have to make plans
- What to expect during the first 24–48 hours post-discharge
- Need to be informed on how to manage pain and discomfort and methods of relieving same
- Increase patients awareness as to the degree of immobility that might be expected; provided patients have this information in advance they can generally cope very well
- Post-operative fatigue, nausea and vomiting
- Eating and drinking
- Elimination
- Ability to drive
- Alcohol intake
- What to do in case of emergency and in the event of complications
- Provide contact number
- Follow up telephone call

offered the opportunity to attend a pre-admission clinic during which time they can receive in-depth information and education on their surgical procedure.

There are day surgery facilities which offer the service of a pre-admission clinic but focus solely on assessing the suitability of patients for day surgery. In some instances patients are assessed for their suitability and simply sent home with written information materials. Thus, missing a golden opportunity to actively engage with and educate and inform patients and carers. This is contrary to recommendations made in the 2002 Department of Health *Day Surgery Operational Guide* which suggest that pre-assessment protocols include information on the day surgery experience, so facilitating patients understanding of the surgical procedure they are to undergo and the likely post-operative course. Rhodes et al. (2006) and Richardson-Tench et al. (2005), in systematic reviews of the day surgery literature, note that the pre-admission clinic improved patient outcomes during the peri-operative period and increased patient satisfaction with after-care instructions.

The pre-admission clinic should not just include patients but also persons who will be caring for them in their own home environment. Verbal and written education and information on pre-operative preparation and post-operative advice will enable patients and carers to make suitable arrangements to their home environment and make necessary plans for discharge (Healthcare Commission 2005). It is important to note that education and information is repeated and reinforced during the patient's stay and on their discharge home. Following a visit to the pre-admission clinic, patients and carers will come to understand the important role they have in contributing to the successful outcome of their day surgery.

As previously outlined, there are patients who may never be offered the opportunity of attending a pre-admission clinic. Such patients need written information on the surgical procedure that they are to undergo and also receive information about the day surgery facility (Audit Commission 2001; Healthcare Commission 2005). Information can include directions and layout of the unit, contact details, and what will take place during the admission process. All of this information should be sent in advance of their admission, thus affording them the opportunity to prepare correctly for the procedure and make the necessary preparations for their recovery at home By posting the information in advance the day surgery unit is offering patients the chance to contact the unit if they have any questions or concerns and also to avoid their non-attendance on the day of surgery (Audit Commission 2001).

On the day patients are admitted to the day surgery unit, information previously given to patients needs to be repeated as many, due to anxiety, experience difficulties recalling this information (Box 7.4).

Discharging patients in day surgery units is a very busy period for nurses so there is a need for an organised and coordinated approach. Indeed,

---

Box 7.4   *Education on morning of admission*

Even though this has already been discussed during the pre-admission clinic and in the written materials provided, there is a need to reinforce the following on the morning of admission:

- Admission process
- Inform carers what time they should return to pick up patient
- Inform patient and carer how long someone should stay with patient once discharged
- Sequential order of events
- Details on proposed surgery
- What to expect in operating room
- What to expect during recovery period
- Importance of adequate pain management and need to report pain as early as possible
- What to expect on discharge
- What to expect at home
- Outline required behaviour, likely sensations that patient may experience during their time in day surgery facility

---

planning and preparing for discharge should begin when patients visit the pre-admission clinic (Royal College of Nursing 2004b; Healthcare Commission 2005). As a result, patients and carers know of and make the necessary arrangements for their discharge in advance of their admission to day surgery. For those patients who do not attend such clinics, written information on discharge should be provided in advance of their admission to the day surgery facility.

Discharge information and education which is procedure specific is repeated and reinforced through the provision of additional written instructions to patients and carers (Box 7.5). Importantly, this information needs to address potential issues that may arise during patients' recovery at home. This will enable patients and carers to solve problems as they arise, thus, avoiding the need to seek assistance from the day surgery unit or primary health care providers (Audit Commission 2001).

Follow-up telephone calls post-discharge are also useful tools in the education and support of patients and carers. This call can be made 24 hours post-discharge and provides nursing personnel with the opportunity to audit the patient's experience of day surgery, education and information materials they received and their post operative period at home. It is

> ### Box 7.5   *Discharge education for patients/carers*
>
> Even though this has already been discussed during the pre admission clinic and in the written materials provided there is a need to reinforce the following on discharge:
>
> - Remind patient of possible recovery time needed, need to go home and rest
> - Must be accompanied home
> - Must have supervision of responsible adult for first 24 hours
> - Provide procedure specific information
> - Effect of sedatives on memory and recall, therefore do not make important decisions or sign anything in the first 24 hours
> - Wound care and dressing to be used – given supply
> - Arrangements for dressing renewal and suture removal (if appropriate) – where, when and by whom
> - If wound drain is present (if drainage is minimal) – care of same and when to be removed
> - Patients with POP must be given instructions covering the first 24 hours post op and also instructions on general care
> - Expected outcomes – what to expect – need to be specific
> - Any specific diet instructions
> - Do not drive on return home
> - Do not operate machinery
> - Drugs specific instructions regarding prescribed analgesia, anti emetics or antibiotics; side effects and general information about drugs, when to administer and how to manage pain
> - When to bathe or shower
> - When to resume normal activities
> - Recognition of post operative complications, what not to expect and what to do if they occur; contact telephone numbers for information or for emergency follow up
> - Telephone follow up services
> - Follow up OPD appointment
> - Other support mechanism is community services GP public health nurse/district health nurse

important that patients give their consent to follow-up telephone calls prior to their discharge, as some may not wish to be followed up. Integrated pathways offer a structured approach to follow-up telephone calls (Box 7.6).

Box 7.6   *Integrated care pathway post-discharge telephone service*
(Aspen Reference Group 1997; St Finbar's Day Ward, Beaumont Hospital, Dublin 2007)

Date of Call: _____   Time: _____   Phone Number: _____

Surgical Procedure: _____

Date of procedure: _____   Surgeon: _____

1   Any problems since your discharge?   ☐ Yes   ☐ No
    (if yes comment)

2   Is your pain   ☐ severe   ☐ moderate   ☐ slight   ☐ none

3   Have you take any pain medication?   ☐ Yes   ☐ No
    (if yes state name of analgesia)
    Was it helpful?   ☐ Yes   ☐ No
    Comments _____

4   Any nausea or vomiting?   ☐ Yes   ☐ No

5   Did you receive an information leaflet about your procedure?
                                                ☐ Yes   ☐ No

6   Did you understand it?   ☐ Yes   ☐ No

7   How did you find your stay in the ward?
    Excellent ☐   Satisfactory ☐   Unsatisfactory ☐
    If unsatisfactory, how do you think we could improve our
    service?

8   Do you require any further advice?
                                                ☐ Yes   ☐ No

9   Do you feel the pre-assessment was beneficial?
                                                ☐ Yes   ☐ No

10 If you were having a similar procedure again, would you
    prefer to come back to the day ward or be admitted
    overnight?
    Inpatient ☐   Day-Patient ☐

Signature of Nurse _____ Date: _____ /_____ /_____

Principles of patient education

The principles of patient education are somewhat similar to the nursing process. The education process like the nursing process provides a systematic and logical framework for the provision of education. It also consists of a continuous cycle of four elements: assessment, planning, implementation and evaluation (Rankin et al. 2005; Bastable 2006). Planning and implementation of teaching is based on the assessment of patients learning needs, readiness to learn and learning styles. Redman (1988) suggests that failure to determine the need to learn and not addressing all of the steps of the education process may impact negatively on the practice, effectiveness and outcomes of patient education.

Assessment phase

As previously stated the education process for day surgery patient should ideally start during the patient's visit to the pre-admission clinic. It also takes place on admission to and discharge from the day surgery unit. The education process begins with the assessment phase. This phase highlights what patients and carers already know and identifies gaps in patients knowledge, their readiness to learn and learning styles.

Assessing learning needs

Within the literature, the term 'education need' is used interchangeably with learning needs and information needs (Falvo 2004). A learning need is described as a gap between what someone knows and what they need to know. This gap may be due to a lack of knowledge, attitude or skills (Bastable 2006). Learning needs can be identified by either the patient or the nurse. However, learning needs identified by nurses need to presented in such a manner that patients will recognise their importance. Failure to do so will result in patients not engaging in the education process. Bastable (2006) identified a number of important elements to the assessment of learning needs:

- Identify the learner
- Choose the right setting
- Collect important information about the learner
- Involve members of the healthcare team
- Prioritise needs
- Time management
- Methods to assess learning needs

Identify the learner

Day surgery nurses at the beginning of the assessment process need to identify who their audience will be. Do you teach a group of patients together and who may or may not be having similar procedures? Will their learning needs be similar or different? If you decide on group teaching, what impact will this have on the day patients desire for individualised information? Once you have identified the learner you need to identify possible teaching opportunities, for instance, will it be formal or informal? Some healthcare settings may have formal, structured educational packages to guide the delivery of education in the day surgery setting, others may have a less structured approach.

Choose the right setting

The visit to the pre-admission clinic needs to be carefully planned in order to make it conducive to learning. Patients should be seen in a private room without fear of interruption and feel secure enough to provide information that is confidential and which may be of an embarrassing nature. The environment needs to be such that nurses recognise this meeting as an ideal opportunity to get to know patients and develop a therapeutic relationship with them. It is important to minimise external distractions, for example, patients referred to the clinic from an outpatients department may not have accounted for this visit in their agenda and subsequently are in a hurry to return home. It may be necessary to rearrange a visit to a time that is more suitable and less distracting for the patient.

Collect important information about the learner

During the pre-admission interview, nurses need to collect information on patients. This information will determine what issues in relation to the procedure and the day surgery experience are important to patients. It is also important to determine what information patients already know about the procedure. What issues do patients need clarified or expanded? This knowledge will facilitate the process of identifying how much and what type of information patients would like to receive. Information on the type of social support patients currently have at home and will have prior to and following their admission for day surgery is also identified. All of this data will determine the extent and content to be included in teaching. It will also assist in identifying the teaching methods and tools that best suit patients and carers. This reflects a patient-centred approach to education. By engaging patients and carers in the education process, nurses are motivating patients to become actively involved in their learning.

Involve members of the healthcare team

Depending on the surgical procedure, there may be a need to be collaborative with other members of the multidisciplinary team. Members of the team may already know the patient and can contribute to the overall planning and delivery of teaching. For teaching and information giving to be consistent, it is also important relevant members of the team are involved in the education process.

Prioritise needs

Prioritising needs is the most challenging area of teaching and has to be agreed between patients and day surgery nurses. Once agreed realistic and achievable learning goals can then be set. It is during this process that patients and nurses agree to the areas that need to be learned and in what depth.

Time management

Adequate time should be set aside for the pre-admission visit so that patients can feel relaxed and not rushed. Patients should be offered the opportunity to actively engage in the education process. The assessment interview typically lasts approximately 20–25 minutes and includes not only the provision of education but also the patient's physical and social assessment. It is, therefore, important that this assessment is carried out by an experienced day surgery nurse who can ascertain fundamental issues that need to be taught to the patient in a very short time, through the use of key, pertinent questions. It must also be remembered that when patients are admitted for day surgery, lack of time can become an issue and so any teaching done at that point should ideally be repeating and reinforcing what patients have already received in the pre-admission clinic or via written materials distributed to them prior to admission.

Methods to assess learning needs

Learning needs can be assessed through the use of causal conversation which requires the use of excellent communications skills. These skills are similar to those identified in the communications chapter of this book. Structured interviews, questionnaires, observations and patient charts are examples of strategies that can be used to assist in the identification of patient learning needs.

Assessing readiness to learn

Readiness to learn refers to when patients are interested in learning information necessary to maintain their health and is willing and able to participate in the education process. If the patient is not ready, then information will not be processed. Bastable (2006) describes four types of readiness to learn, which we have applied to the day surgery setting:

- Physical Readiness
- Emotional Readiness
- Experiential Readiness
- Knowledge Readiness.

Physical readiness

There are a number of components to physical readiness which include measures of ability, complexity of task, environmental effects and health status. During the visit to the pre-admission clinic, nurses need to determine if any of these factors are relevant to patients that they are assessing. For example, when assessing for measures of ability the nurse is seeking out any information on the patient's physical ability that may impact on the education process such as eye impairment. This may require the use of audiotapes instead of providing written materials to patients. If there is no audiotape available then it is imperative that carers are present throughout the period that information is provided to patients. Written material also needs to be explained and given to carers.

There is also a need to determine the complexity of the information being giving to patients and whether this will be difficult to master. For example, patients may be required to instil eye drops prior to their admission and may find this skill too complex, resulting in their reluctance to engage in teaching. Environmental readiness is linked to creating an environment that is conducive to learning and ensuring that teaching activities are well paced to suit the needs of the learner. Health status relates to the amount of energy needed by the patient to learn. If patients have acute or chronic pain then they may have little energy to learn.

Emotional readiness

In order to determine how emotionally ready a patient is to learn, a number of areas need to be assessed, including anxiety level, support systems and motivation.

Anxiety influences patients' ability to carry out physical and mental tasks which may impact on their ability to learn. Day surgery patients' fears may also impact negatively on their readiness to learn. Consequently, there is a need to repeat information both on admission to the day surgery facility and at discharge. The degree of anxiety experienced may also be linked to the support systems available to the patient. A strong support system will influence the emotional readiness of the patient to learn. Those patients whose support system is not strong will need greater support from staff in the day surgery unit. Indeed, day surgery may not be an option for those patients who have no support systems in place. Determining the level of motivation is also linked to emotional readiness. Patients who show an interest or ask questions are ready to learn. Many patients attending day surgery are motivated to learn by the prospect of not having to stay over-night in hospital.

Experiential readiness

There is a need to assess patients' previous learning experiences within the healthcare system. A negative experience may result in unmotivated patients who are unwilling to engage in the education process. This is also the opportunity to identify patients coping styles and determine if they avoidant or vigilant copers. From this information, nurses can determine the level of information to give patients.

Day surgery nurses also need to be aware of other cultures and their beliefs in relation to illness and education. Using this knowledge can assist nurses in determining patients' readiness to learn. Difficulties in language may necessitate the use of an interpreter during patients visit to the pre-admission clinic and their admission to the day surgery unit.

Knowledge readiness

Knowledge readiness refers to the present knowledge base, learning capability and preferred learning style of patients. This involves identifying what patients and carers already know about the procedure and what is required of them when caring for themselves at home. During this process it is important to determine the cognitive ability of patients, identify any learning disabilities and what level of reading skills they possess. This information will shape the approach nurses take to teaching patients. For example, patients with poor cognitive ability or learning disabilities will require instructions to be broken down into simple steps which will need to be repeated.

Assessing how someone learns best (learning style) will help the day nurses select teaching approaches, methods and materials that patients will tolerate. For example, does the patient prefer one-to-one teaching or group teaching? Does the patient prefer reading or viewing a video?

Planning and implementing teaching

Information gathered during the assessment phase will determine the design of a teaching plan. This plan should address the individual learning needs of patients and include goals and expected outcomes. Decisions need to be made by day surgery nurses on the sequence of events, the teaching methods to be used and the resources needed to implement this plan (Box 7.7).

Box 7.7   *Teaching methods and teaching resources*

Teaching Methods:

- Lecture
- Group discussion
- One-to-one teaching
- Demonstration and return demonstration
- Incremental, repeated and reinforced teaching supplemented with written information

Teaching Resources:

- Written materials (handouts, leaflets, pre admission booklets, books, pamphlets, brochures, and instruction sheets
- Commercially prepared materials (posters, pamphlets, brochures and instruction sheets)
- Demonstration materials (models, real equipment, displays – poster, diagrams, photographs, charts, physical objects)
- Audio visual aids (dependent on available resources)
    - audio visual projection equipment
    - use power point presentations
    - overhead projector
    - use of transparencies
    - video projected onto screen
    - video tapes
    - compact disc video
    - radio
    - telecommunications – television and telephone
    - pre-admission and post-discharge follow up telephone call
- pre-admission visit
- information folder in waiting room of day surgery preferable on bedside locker
- use of interpreters
- multidisciplinary involvement
- useful web sites

However, these decisions will be influenced by the financial resources available within the local health care setting. Limited finances will impact on the availability of audio visual equipment and the professional printing of written materials.

Implementation of the teaching plan involves being flexible and responsive to the needs of patients. Teaching should be incremental with emphasis placed on important points. Indeed, key points need to be recapped regularly during the delivery of the educational content. Language needs to be free of medical jargon: it must be concise, clear and appropriate for the intended audience. If medical jargon is used, it needs to explained and patients' understanding evaluated. Teaching may be supported through the use of visual aids such as diagrams or pictures. Throughout the teaching session, patient and carer participation is encouraged by providing time for questions and clarification. Teaching is supported by the use of written materials whose content and layout are explained to patients and carers. These materials can be used as a resource for patients when at home in their own environment.

Evaluation

The final component of the education process is an evaluation of the effectiveness of education and determines the extent to which teaching and learning has been successful (Bastable 2006). Evaluation of teaching and learning needs to be structured and planned. It involves the collection of data through observation, interview, questionnaires or follow up telephone calls.

Within day surgery, the effectiveness of education can be determined on the day of admission. Patients who present themselves for surgery as per the education they received clearly demonstrate the effectiveness of that education. On the other hand, patients may attend inappropriately prepared: for example, they may not have fasted or have no responsible adult available to collect them on discharge. The education process has clearly failed this group of patients. In addition, if a unit experiences a high number of 'did not attends', this could call into question the effectiveness of its education programme and the provision of written information material. The continuous use of audits within the day surgery unit will identify these weaknesses within the system. The follow-up telephone also contributes to the evaluation process.

Developing written information material

A patient's visit to the pre-admission clinic is an intense period during which they are required to assimilate a large volume of information within a very short timeframe. This is also apparent when patients are discharged from the day surgery unit. It is clearly evident from the research literature that a larger percentage of information giving during both of these periods is not retained (Law 1997; Moult et al. 2004). Consequently, there is a need to supplement verbal instructions with the provision of written materials. These materials can be read by patients and carers in their own time in their home environment, and can be used as a reference guide for any concerns that may arise during the pre-admission or post-discharge stage of their journey through day surgery. But in order for written instructions to be effective they must meet the needs of their intended audience.

A structured plan needs to be put into place when producing written information. Firstly, the need for specific written material needs to be identified and this is informed by the day surgery patient population. Once the focus and purpose of the written material is identified, a decision needs to be made as to how this process will be coordinated. For example, will it be lead by the nurse manager of the day surgery unit? Following this, the local policy on the development and printing of written information material needs to be examined. Before starting the long process of developing these materials it is useful to check if other departments or nearby day surgery units have produced similar material. If so, then these could be adapted to your own health care setting. Once this information has been gathered, the next stage is to establish a development group.

The development group consists of representatives from all key stakeholders in day surgery, including patient groups. Involving representatives from the patient population will enable the development team to identify what information patients would find useful. However, there are also a number of considerations to be made before producing the first draft of the written material (Box 7.8).

Written material must be easy to read. The readability of material is determined by the degree to which it matches the patients reading skills or levels (Tutty and O'Connor 1999). Many people read at a level that is below their completed formal education (Mitchell 2001; Brown 2006). This has implications for developing written material, as it needs to be pitched at a level that is easily understood by patients. Moult et al. (2004) suggest that written material which reflects low reading levels is more likely to be read and understood by a larger proportion of the public. Indeed, material that does not reflect patients' cognitive level or reading level will not be read and prove to be uneconomical and worthless.

In many day surgery units, patients receive a generic admission booklet and a procedure specific leaflet or information sheet. The content of all day surgery written material needs to reflect the verbal instructions given to patients at the pre-admission clinic, on day of admission and at discharge (Boxes 7.3, 7.4, 7.5). These materials should include both procedure and sensory information. The front page of any written material needs to clearly indicate its focus and purpose, therefore, its title needs to be clear and

Box 7.8   Developing written materials *(National Health Promotion Unit 2003; NHS 2003; the Basic Skills Agency 2005; the British Dyslexia Association 2007; National Adult Literacy Agency 2007)*

For written material to be comprehensible and easy to read:

- Sentences need to be simple and short
- Sentences should have no more than 15–20 words
- Words used should be no more that three syllabus long
- Sentences should include no more than one idea
- Personalise written material by using personal nouns ('you' and 'we') – the use of these terms will make the patient feel that the material is talking to them
- Use present tense and active voice when structuring sentences ('your appointment is on' or 'you are required to attend on')
- Use everyday language
- Avoid the use of jargon, slang or inaccurate expressions ('you will be put to sleep' instead use 'general anaesthetic')
- If medical terms are to be used, they need to be explained immediately within the text
- Avoid the use of abbreviations

Layout of written material:

- Can use the format of frequently asked questions or list of 'do's and don'ts'
- The minimum font type size to be used is size 12
- Use a sans serif type face such as Arial, Verdana Helvetica or Tahoma
- Use of bold to highlight content should be used minimally
- Do not use italic font style or underline text
- Captions should be in lower case (capitals are less distinct, difficult to read and result in patients not reading information)
- Avoid sentences written entirely in capitals
- Leave spacing between lines (this will leave white space allowing the reader to navigate their way around the text)
- Avoid dense blocks of text
- Use shorter paragraphs
- Use bullet points to break up important information
- Pages should have margins of 2cm (patients experience difficulty reading text on pages with no margins)
- Avoid writing text over background pictures, designs or against a dark background
- Appropriate illustrations can be incorporated into the written material (increase patients understanding of a procedure)
- Preferred printing paper should matt finish (avoid glossy paper)

concise. A department logo also needs to be placed on the front page, so helping patients to identify the unit. Space needs to be provided on the front cover to allow for the insertion of the patient's name and the date and time of their admission to the day surgery unit. It is recommended that the back page should include a location map of the day surgery unit, the date of publication, address and contact details of department, leaflet code, organisation copyright and its web site address (NHS 2003).

The first draft of the written material needs to be distributed to all key stakeholders who are expected to provide feedback within a given timeframe. The content needs to be checked for accuracy ensuring that it is not in conflict with any other information. Contact telephone details included in the material also need to checked. When final editing is complete, it is important at this stage to pilot test the written material with the relevant patient group. This group needs to provide feedback on the readability of the material, its suitability and if it addressed their concerns. Once this is complete, the final document can be then sent to the printer but the printer's proofs needs to be checked before final printing.

Conclusion

Further expansion of day surgery services is dependent on the self-care abilities of patients and carers. It is also dependent on their willingness to actively engage and manage their own recovery. The ongoing provision of both verbal and written information to patients and carers is essential to the continued success of this service. Underpinning this success is the need for day surgery nurses to have a full understanding and appreciation of the education process. The provision of verbal and written information is continuously evolving, with many day surgery units exploring new technologies to assist them in this process. The advancement of the World Wide Web is one such resource that needs to be harnessed by day surgery facility and put to effective use in the education of patients and carers. This could involve patients accessing a specific web site from home and downloading computer-generated, individualised instructions. Other areas that need to be further developed are formalised procedure-specific educational packages and development of post-discharge help lines. Ultimately, involvement of patients and carers in the education process is the cornerstone to a successful and effective day surgery service.

References

Aspen Reference Group (1997) *Ambulatory Surgery: Patient Education Manual.* Aspen Publication, Gaitherburg, Maryland.

Association of Anaesthetists of Great Britain and Ireland (AAGBI) (2005) *Day Surgery*, revised edn. AAGBI, London.

Audit Commission (2001) *Acute Hospital Portfolio, Review of National Findings, Day Surgery*. Audit Commission, London.

Audit Commission for Local Authorities and the National Health Service in England and Wales (1990) *A Short Cut to Better Services: Day Surgery in England and Wales*. HMSO, London.

Bastable, S. (2006) *Essentials of Patient Education*. Jones and Bartlett Publishers, Boston.

Basic Skills Agency (2005) *Readability: How to Produce Clear Written Materials for a Range of Readers*, The Basic Skills Agency, London.

British Dyslexia Association (2007) *Dyslexia Style Guide*. The British Dyslexia Association, London.

Bernier, M., Sanares, D., Owen, S. and Newhouse, P. (2003) Preoperative teaching received and valued in a day surgery setting. *Association of Operating Room Nurses, AORN Journal*, 77(3), 563–82.

Boore, J. (1978) *Prescription for Recovery*, Royal College of Nurses, London.

Brown, V. (2006) Preparing a patient information leaflet. *Journal of Perioperative Practice*, 16(11), 540–45.

Butler, M., Treacy, M., Scott, A., Hyde, A., Mac Neela, P. Irving, K., Byrne, A. and Drennan, J. (2006) Towards a nursing minimum data set for Ireland: Making Irish nursing visible. *Journal of Advanced Nursing*, 55(3), 364–75.

Costa, M. (2001) The lived perioperative experience of ambulatory surgery patients. *Association of Operating Room Nurses, AORN Journal*, 74(6), 874–81.

Cox, H. and O'Connell, B. (2003) Recovery from gynaecological day surgery: Are we underestimating the process? *Journal of Ambulatory Surgery*, 14, 114–21.

Department of Health (2000) *The NHS Plan: A Plan for Investment, a Plan for Reform*, Department of Health, London.

Department of Health (2002) *Day Surgery: Operational Guide: Waiting, Booking and Choice*, Department of Health, London.

Devine, E. and Cook, T. (1986) Clinical and cost saving effects of psycho-educational interventions with surgical patients: A meta analysis. *Research in Nursing and Health*, 9, 89–105.

Dewar, A., Craig, K., Muir, J. and Cole, C. (2003) Testing the effectiveness of a nursing intervention in relieving pain following day surgery. *Journal of Ambulatory Surgery*, 10, 81–8.

Falvo, D. (2004) *Effective Patient Education: A Guide to Increased Compliance*, Jones and Bartlett Publishers, Sudbury.

Grieve, R. (2002) Day surgery preoperative anxiety reduction and coping strategies. *British Journal of Nursing*, 11(10), 670–8.

Hayward, J. (1975) *Information: A Prescription Against Pain*. Royal College of Nursing, London.

Healthcare Commission (2005) *Day Surgery: Acute Hospital Portfolio Review*, Healthcare Commission, London.

Howard, J., Davies, J. and Roghmann, K. (1987) Respiratory teaching of patients: How effective is it? *Journal of Advanced Nursing*, 12(2), 207–14.

Law, M. (1997) A telephone survey of day-surgery eye patients. *Journal of Advanced Nursing*, 25, 355–63.

Majasaari, H., Sarajarvi, A., Koskinen, H., Autere, S. and Paavilainen, E. (2005) Patients' perceptions of emotional support and information provided to family members. *AORN Journal*, 81(5), 1030–9.

McHugh, G. and Thoms, G. (2002) The management of pain following day-case surgery. *Anaesthesia*, 57, 266–83.

Mitchell, M. (1997) Patients' perceptions of post-operative preparation for day surgery. *Journal of Advanced Nursing*, 26, 356–63.

Mitchell, M. (2000) Anxiety management: A distinct nursing role in day surgery. *Journal of Ambulatory Surgery*, 8, 119–27.

Mitchell, M. (2000a) Psychological preparation for patients undergoing day surgery. *Journal of Ambulatory Surgery*, 8, 19–29.

Mitchell, M. (2001) Constructing information booklets for day case patients. *Ambulatory Surgery*, 9, 37–45.

Mitchell, M. (2002) Guidance for the psychological care of day case surgery patients. *Nursing Standard*, 16(40), 41–3.

Mitchell, M. (2005) *Anxiety management in adult day surgery: a nursing perspective*, Whurr, London.

Mottram, A. (2001) Pre-registration student nurses' perceptions of the day surgery unit. *Journal of Ambulatory Surgery*, 9, 103–107.

Moult, B., Franck, L. and Brady, H. (2004) Ensuring quality information for patients: development and preliminary validation of a new instrument to improve the quality of written health care information. *Health Expectations*, 7, 165–75.

National Adult Literacy Agency (2007) *Writing and Design Tips*, National Adult Literacy Agency. http://www.nala.ie, Dublin (accessed December 2007).

National Health Promotion Unit (2003) *Writing Effective Health Information Materials, Guidelines on writing and design technique*, National Health Promotion Unit, Dublin.

National Health Service (2003) *Toolkit for Producing Patient Information*, Department of Health, London.

Otte, D. (1996) Patients' perspectives and experiences of day case surgery. *Journal of Advanced Nursing*, 23, 1228–37.

Pearson, A., Richardson, M. and Cairns, M. (2004) 'Best Practice' in day surgery units: A review of the evidence. *Journal of Ambulatory Surgery*, 11, 49–54.

Rankin, S., Stallings, K. and London, F. (Eds.) (2005) *Patient Education in Health and Illness*, Lippincott Williams & Wilkins, Philadelphia.

Redman, B. (1988) *The Process of Patient Education*, 6th edn. CV Mosby Company, St Louis.

Redman, B. (2004) *Advances in Patient Education*, Springer Publishing Company, New York.

Rhodes, L., Miles, G. and Pearson, A. (2006) Patient subjective experience and satisfaction during the perioperative period in the day surgery setting: A systematic review. *International Journal of Nursing Practice*, 12, 178–92.

Richardson-Tench, M., Pearson, A. and Birks, M. (2005) The changing face of sugery using systematic reviews. *British Journal of Perioperative Nursing*, 15(6), 240–6.

Royal College of Nursing (2004b) *Day Surgery Information, Discharge Planning*, Royal College of Nursing, London.

St Finbars Day Ward Beaumont Hospital Dublin (2007) *Pre-operative and Post-Operative Patient Record for General Anaesthetics*. Beaumont Hospital, Dublin.

Tutty, L. and O'Connor, G. (1999) Patient information leaflets: Some pertinent guidelines. *Radiography*, 5(1), 11–14.

Twersky, R., Fishman, D. and Homel, P. (1997) What happens after discharge? Return hospital visits after ambulatory surgery. *Anaesthesia Analgesia*, 84, 319–24.

Watt-Watson, J., Chung, F., Chan, V., McGillion, M. (2004) Pain management following discharge after ambulatory same-day surgery. *Journal of Nursing Management*, 12, 153–61.

Wilson-Barnett, J. (1978) Patients emotional responses to Barium X-rays. *Journal of Advanced Nursing*, 3(1), 37–46.

Wilson-Barnett, J. and Osbourne, J. (1983) Studies evaluating patient teaching: Implications for practice. *International Journal of Nursing Studies*, 20(1), 33–44.

Young, J., O'Connell, B. and McGregor, S. (2000) Day surgery patients' convalescences at home: Does enhanced discharge education make a difference? *Nursing and Health Sciences*, 2, 29–39.

Index

Note: page numbers in *italics* refer to figures, those in **bold** refer to tables and boxes